ACKNOWLEDGEMENT

Writing this eBook has been a journey of discovery, learning, and immense growth. It is with deep gratitude that I acknowledge the many individuals and groups whose support, encouragement, and guidance made this project possible.

First and foremost, I would like to thank my family for their unwavering support and patience throughout this process. Your belief in me provided the motivation I needed to see this project through to completion. Thank you for understanding the late nights, the time spent researching and writing, and for always being my strongest pillars of support.

I would also like to express my heartfelt thanks to my friends, who offered their encouragement, feedback, and constant reminders to stay focused and committed. Your words of wisdom and thoughtful insights were instrumental in shaping this book into what it is today.

To the healthcare professionals, nutritionists, and experts in the field of diabetes management who generously shared their knowledge, I am deeply indebted. Your expertise and guidance were crucial in ensuring that the information presented in this eBook is accurate, practical, and beneficial for those who are managing diabetes after 50.

A special note of appreciation goes to the community of individuals living with diabetes who shared their stories, challenges, and successes with me. Your experiences provided invaluable perspectives that enriched the content of this book, making it more relatable and useful for readers.

I would also like to thank the editorial and design team, whose dedication to this project ensured that the final product is not only informative but also engaging and accessible. Your meticulous attention to detail and creative input have been key in bringing this book to life.

Lastly, to the readers of this eBook, I extend my deepest gratitude. Your trust in this book as a resource for managing diabetes means the world to me. It is my sincere hope that the recipes and advice within these pages will serve as a valuable tool in your journey to a healthier, happier life.

Thank you all for being a part of this journey with me.

— Dr. Mark B. Atkins

PREFACE

Welcome to "Easy Diabetic Diet Recipes After 50: Low Sugar, Low Carb recipes for Type 1 and Type 2 Diabetes including Weekly Meal Plans for Healthier Life."

As a Registered Dietitian Nutritionist with extensive experience in clinical nutrition and a deep understanding of diabetes management, I have dedicated my career to helping individuals achieve optimal health through dietary modifications. My journey in this field has been shaped by my interactions with patients, ongoing research, and a commitment to improving quality of life through effective nutrition strategies.

This eBook was inspired by the growing need for accessible, practical resources tailored to individuals over 50 who are managing diabetes. Throughout my career, I've observed how complex and overwhelming it can be to navigate dietary restrictions while trying to maintain a satisfying and healthy diet. I wanted to create a resource that simplifies this process, offering delicious and nutritious recipes that align with low sugar and low carb guidelines.

The primary objective of this eBook is to provide a comprehensive collection of low sugar, low carb recipes specifically crafted for those managing diabetes after 50. Each recipe is designed to be not only health-conscious but also enjoyable, making it easier to adhere to dietary guidelines without sacrificing flavor. I aim to empower readers with the knowledge and tools needed to make informed food choices and to inspire a more balanced approach to eating.

To make the most of this eBook, start by familiarizing yourself with the 'Getting Started' section, which outlines the fundamental principles of managing diabetes through diet. The recipes are organized into categories such as breakfast, lunch, dinner, snacks, and desserts, making it easy to find options that suit any meal or occasion. Use the meal planning tips to integrate these recipes into your weekly routine, and refer to the additional resources section for further support and guidance.

I would like to extend my sincere thanks to my family, friends, and colleagues whose support and encouragement have been instrumental in bringing this book to fruition. Your belief in this project has been a constant source of motivation.

I hope you find this eBook to be a valuable resource on your journey to better health. Remember, managing diabetes is a continuous process, and making dietary changes can lead to significant improvements in your well-being. I am excited for you to explore these recipes and incorporate them into your daily life. Here's to a healthier, more vibrant you!

Warm regards,

Dr. Mark B. Atkins

Table of Contents

2. Low Carb Chicken Caesar Wrap

3. Mediterranean Tuna Salad

4. Spinach and Mushroom Stuffed Chicken Breast

5. Turkey Lettuce Wraps

6. Cauliflower Rice with Stir-Fried Vegetables

7. Caprese Salad with Balsamic Glaze

8. Beef and Broccoli Stir-Fry

9. Low Carb Vegetable Soup with Chicken

5. **Dinner Recipes**

0. Baked Salmon with Asparagus

1. Stuffed Bell Peppers with Ground Turkey

2. Garlic Butter Steak Bites with Green Beans

3. Low Carb Chicken Parmesan

4. Lemon Herb Roasted Chicken with Brussels Sprouts

5. Grilled Pork Chops with Cauliflower Mash

6. Zoodles with Meatballs in Marinara Sauce

7. Shrimp Scampi with Zucchini Noodles

8. Herb-Crusted Cod with Steamed Broccoli

9. Eggplant Lasagna

6. **Snack Ideas**

0. Almonds and Cheese

1. Cucumber Slices with Hummus

2. Celery Sticks with Peanut Butter

3. Hard-Boiled Eggs with a Dash of Hot Sauce

4. Greek Yogurt with Nuts and Seeds

5. Guacamole with Veggie Sticks

6. Low Carb Cheese Crackers

7. Tuna Salad Lettuce Boats

8. Deviled Eggs

9. Roasted Pumpkin Seeds

7. **Desserts**

0. Chia Seed Pudding

1. Dark Chocolate and Almond Bark

2. Keto Cheesecake Bites

3. Sugar-Free Gelatin with Whipped Cream

4. Coconut Macaroons

5. Low Carb Lemon Bars

6. Almond Flour Brownies

7. Berry Compote with Greek Yogurt

8. Chocolate Avocado Mousse

9. Peanut Butter Fat Bombs

8. **Meal Planning Tips**

- Creating a Weekly Meal Plan

- Batch Cooking and Freezing

GETTING STARTED

Embarking on a journey to manage diabetes effectively involves understanding how to adjust your diet and lifestyle. This section is designed to lay the groundwork for a successful transition to a healthier way of eating and living. We will cover three main areas to help you get started: understanding diabetes after 50, the importance of a low sugar, low carb diet, and how to use this book effectively.

Understanding Diabetes After 50

Diabetes and Aging

As we age, our bodies undergo numerous changes that can affect how we manage chronic conditions like diabetes. For individuals over 50, managing diabetes can become more complex due to a combination of factors such as decreased insulin sensitivity, changes in metabolism, and the presence of other age-related health conditions. Understanding these changes is crucial for effective diabetes management.

Types of Diabetes

1. **Type 2 Diabetes**: This is the most common form of diabetes in older adults. It often develops due to a combination of genetic and lifestyle factors. With Type 2 diabetes, the body becomes resistant to insulin, leading to elevated blood sugar levels.

2. **Type 1 Diabetes**: Though less common in older adults, Type 1 diabetes can also present after 50. It is an autoimmune condition where the pancreas produces little to no insulin.

Impact of Aging on Diabetes Management

Aging can impact diabetes management in several ways:

- **Insulin Resistance**: As we age, our cells may become more resistant to insulin, making blood sugar control more challenging.

- **Changes in Physical Activity**: Reduced physical activity can affect glucose metabolism and increase the risk of weight gain, which can complicate diabetes management.

- **Medications and Health Conditions**: Older adults often manage multiple health conditions and may take various medications, which can interact with diabetes medications and impact blood sugar control.

Understanding these aspects helps tailor dietary and lifestyle interventions that address the unique needs of older adults managing diabetes.

The Importance of Low Sugar, Low Carb Diets

Managing Blood Sugar Levels

A low sugar, low carb diet is crucial for managing diabetes, particularly for those over 50. Here's why:

- **Blood Sugar Control**: Reducing carbohydrate intake helps to lower blood sugar levels and prevent spikes. Carbohydrates are broken down into glucose, which can raise blood sugar levels if not managed properly.

- **Insulin Sensitivity**: Lowering sugar and carb intake can improve insulin sensitivity, which is essential for effective blood sugar management.

- **Weight Management**: A diet low in sugar and carbs can help in maintaining a healthy weight, which is important for diabetes control.

Health Benefits

- **Reduced Risk of Complications**: A low sugar, low carb diet can lower the risk of diabetes-related complications such as cardiovascular disease, neuropathy, and retinopathy.

- **Improved Energy Levels**: Consuming fewer sugars and carbs can help stabilize energy levels throughout the day, preventing the fatigue and energy crashes associated with high sugar intake.

- **Enhanced Overall Health**: This type of diet can contribute to better heart health, improved digestion, and a lower risk of other chronic diseases.

Adapting Your Diet

Transitioning to a low sugar, low carb diet involves making mindful food choices, focusing on nutrient-dense foods, and understanding how different foods impact blood sugar levels. This dietary approach emphasizes whole foods like vegetables, lean proteins, and healthy fats while minimizing processed foods, sugary snacks, and refined carbs.

How to Use This Book

Navigating the Content

This eBook is designed to be a practical guide for managing diabetes through diet. Here's how to make the most of it:

- **Start with the Basics**: Begin by reading the 'Getting Started' section to build a foundational understanding of diabetes management and the principles behind a low sugar, low carb diet.

- **Explore Essential Ingredients and Tools**: Familiarize yourself with the essential ingredients and kitchen tools outlined in the book. This will help you stock your kitchen and prepare meals efficiently.

- **Follow the Recipes**: Dive into the recipe sections, which are categorized by meal type. Each recipe is designed to be both diabetes-friendly and delicious, with clear instructions and nutritional information.

- **Utilize Meal Planning Tips**: Refer to the meal planning tips to help you create a weekly meal plan, manage your shopping, and incorporate the recipes into your daily routine.

- **Leverage Additional Resources**: Use the additional resources section for further support, including recommended books, websites, support groups, and apps.

Making Dietary Changes

Implementing dietary changes can be challenging, but this book is designed to make the process as smooth as possible. Start by integrating a few recipes into your routine and gradually adjust your diet as you become more comfortable. Use the meal planning and shopping tips to streamline the process and make adherence to a low sugar, low carb diet easier.

Tracking Your Progress

Keep track of how the dietary changes impact your blood sugar levels, energy, and overall health. Adjust the recipes and meal plans as needed to fit your personal preferences and nutritional needs. Remember that managing diabetes is an ongoing journey, and making gradual, sustainable changes can lead to long-term success.

CHAPTER 1

ESSENTIAL INGREDIENTS AND TOOLS

Pantry Staples for a Diabetic Kitchen

A well-stocked pantry is the cornerstone of a successful diabetic meal plan. It provides the foundation for creating balanced, low-carb, and low-sugar meals that support optimal blood sugar control and overall health. Below is an in-depth look at essential pantry staples:

Whole Grains and Alternatives

- **Quinoa:**

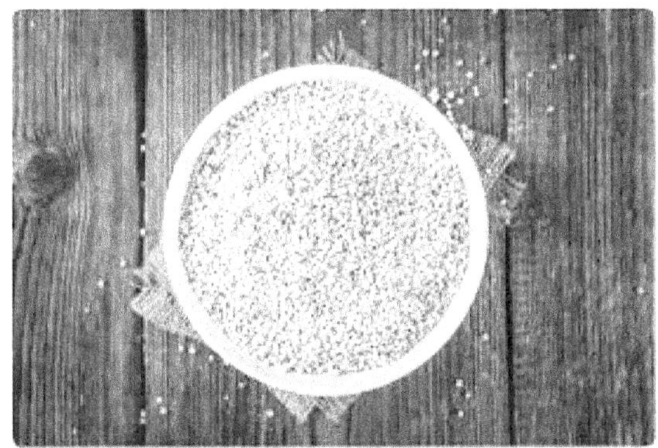

  - **Description:** A versatile, protein-rich grain that is also a complete protein source, making it ideal for vegetarians and those looking to increase protein intake.

  - **Benefits:** High in fiber, which helps to regulate blood sugar levels and improve digestion. It also contains important vitamins and minerals such as magnesium, iron, and B-vitamins.

  - **Uses:** Use quinoa as a base for salads, side dishes, or as a substitute for rice in various recipes.

- **Brown Rice:**

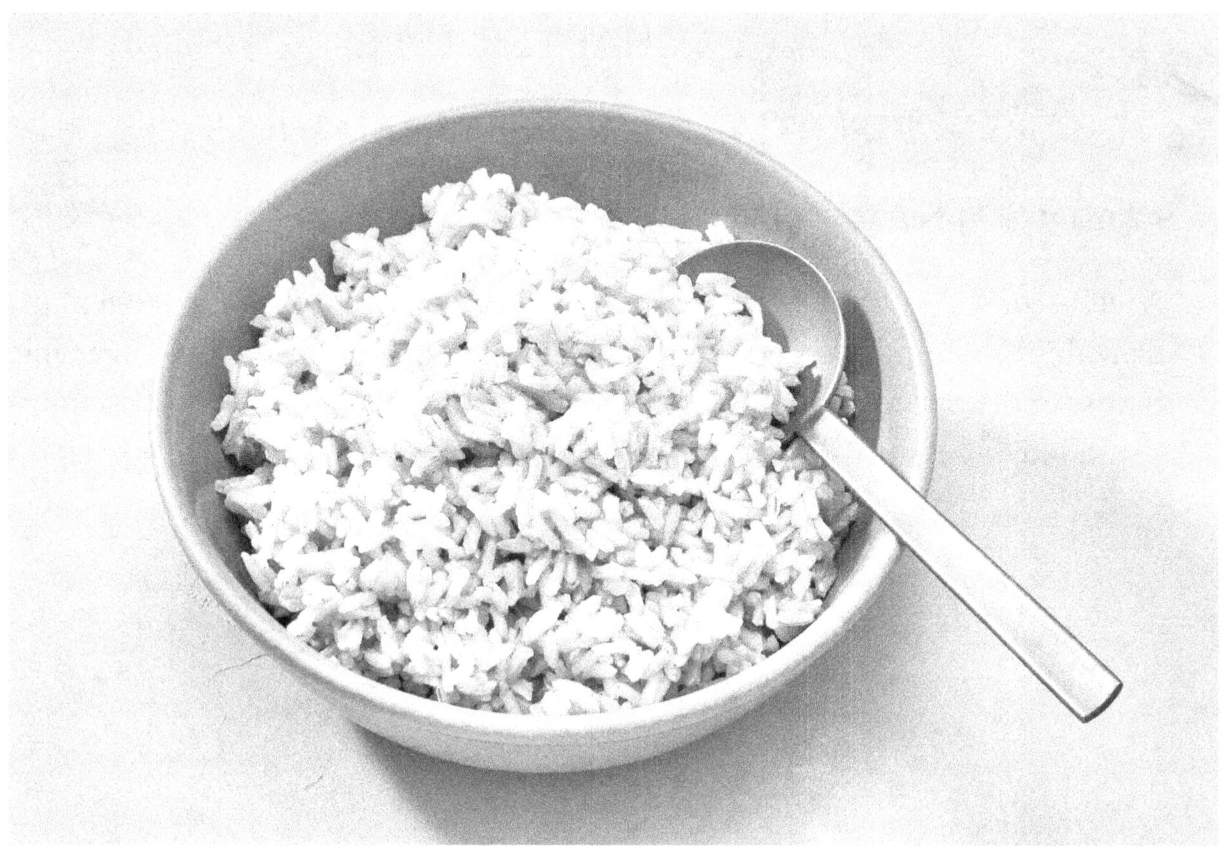

- o **Description:** Less processed than white rice, it retains its bran and germ, providing more fiber and nutrients.

- o **Benefits:** Helps in stabilizing blood sugar levels due to its high fiber content and has a lower glycemic index compared to white rice.

- o **Uses:** Ideal for serving with stir-fries, curries, and as a component in grain bowls.

- **Oats:**

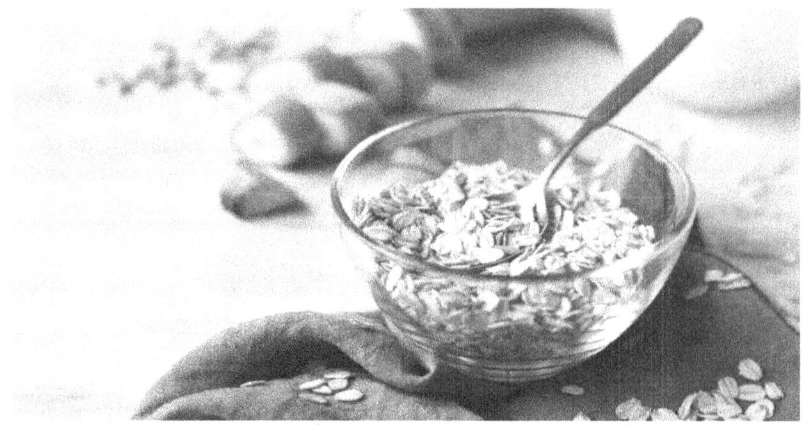

- o **Description:** Whole oats are a great source of soluble fiber, particularly beta-glucan, which has been shown to help lower cholesterol levels.

- o **Benefits:** Supports stable blood sugar levels and provides a slow release of energy.

- o **Uses:** Prepare as oatmeal, add to smoothies, or use in baking low-carb treats.

Legumes

- **Chickpeas:**

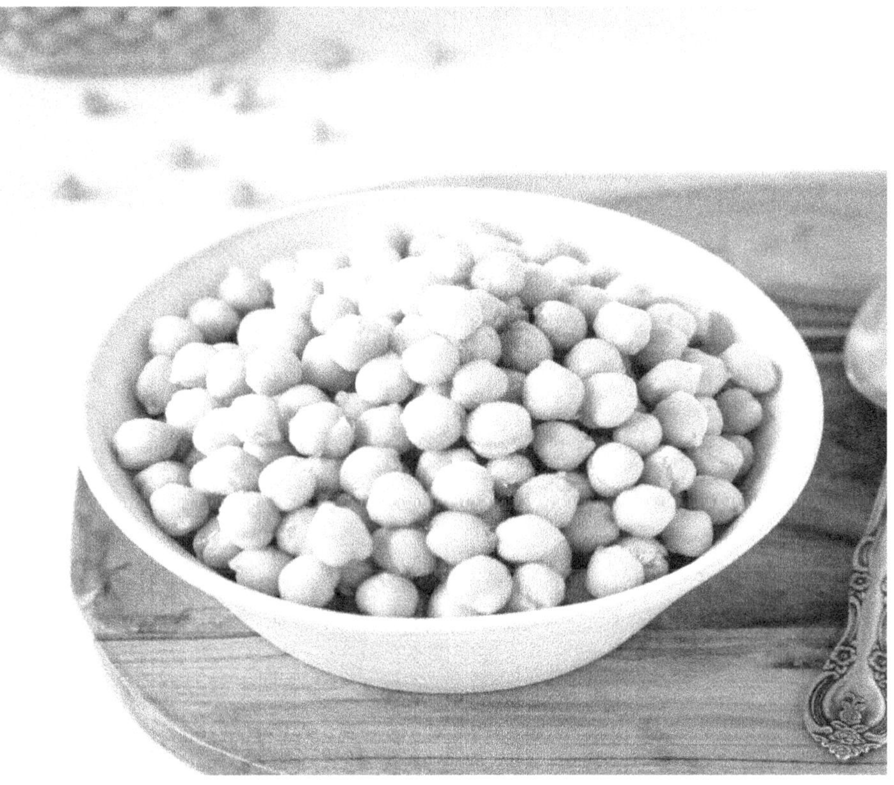

- o **Description:** Also known as garbanzo beans, chickpeas are a staple in many cuisines.

- o **Benefits:** High in protein and fiber, chickpeas help with blood sugar regulation and provide sustained energy.

- ○ **Uses:** Use in salads, soups, or as a base for homemade hummus.

- **Lentils:**

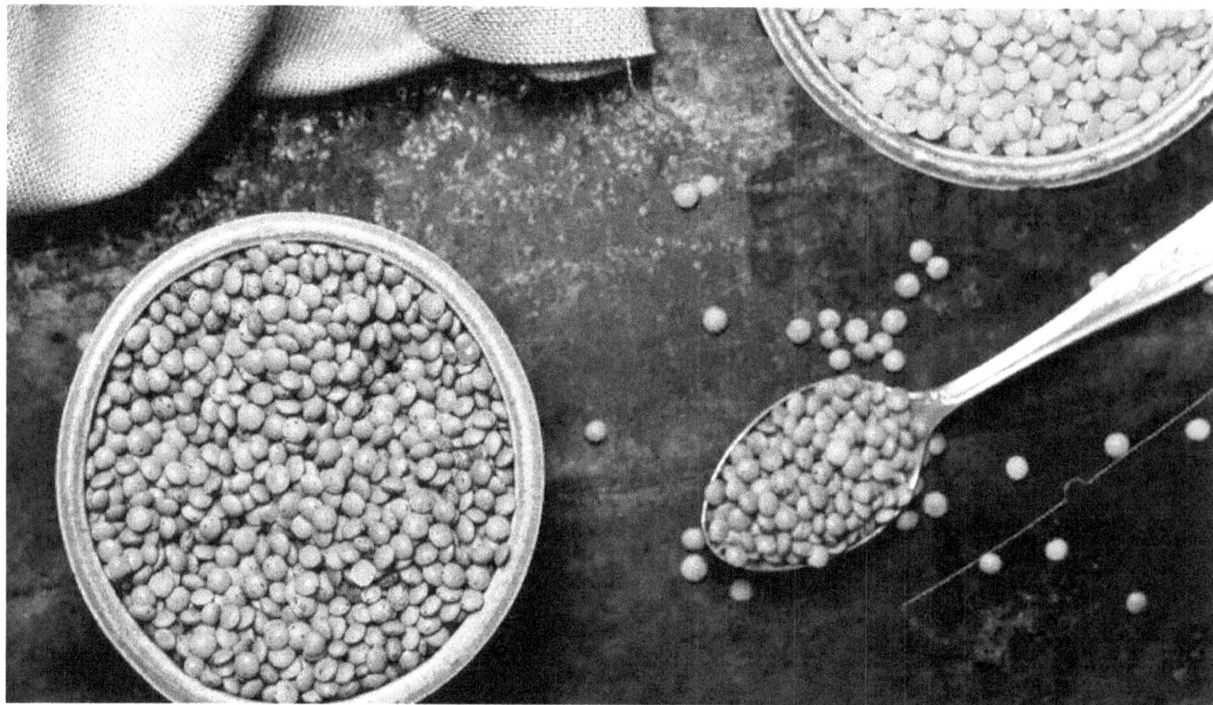

- ○ **Description:** A type of pulse that comes in various colors such as green, brown, and red.

- ○ **Benefits:** Rich in fiber, protein, and essential nutrients. They help with blood sugar control and digestive health.

- ○ **Uses:** Perfect for soups, stews, and salads, or as a meat substitute in vegetarian dishes.

- **Black Beans:**

- ○ **Description:** Small, round beans with a slightly sweet flavor.

- ○ **Benefits:** High in fiber and antioxidants, black beans support blood sugar management and overall heart health.

- ○ **Uses:** Incorporate into salads, soups, or use as a base for chili.

- **Almonds:**

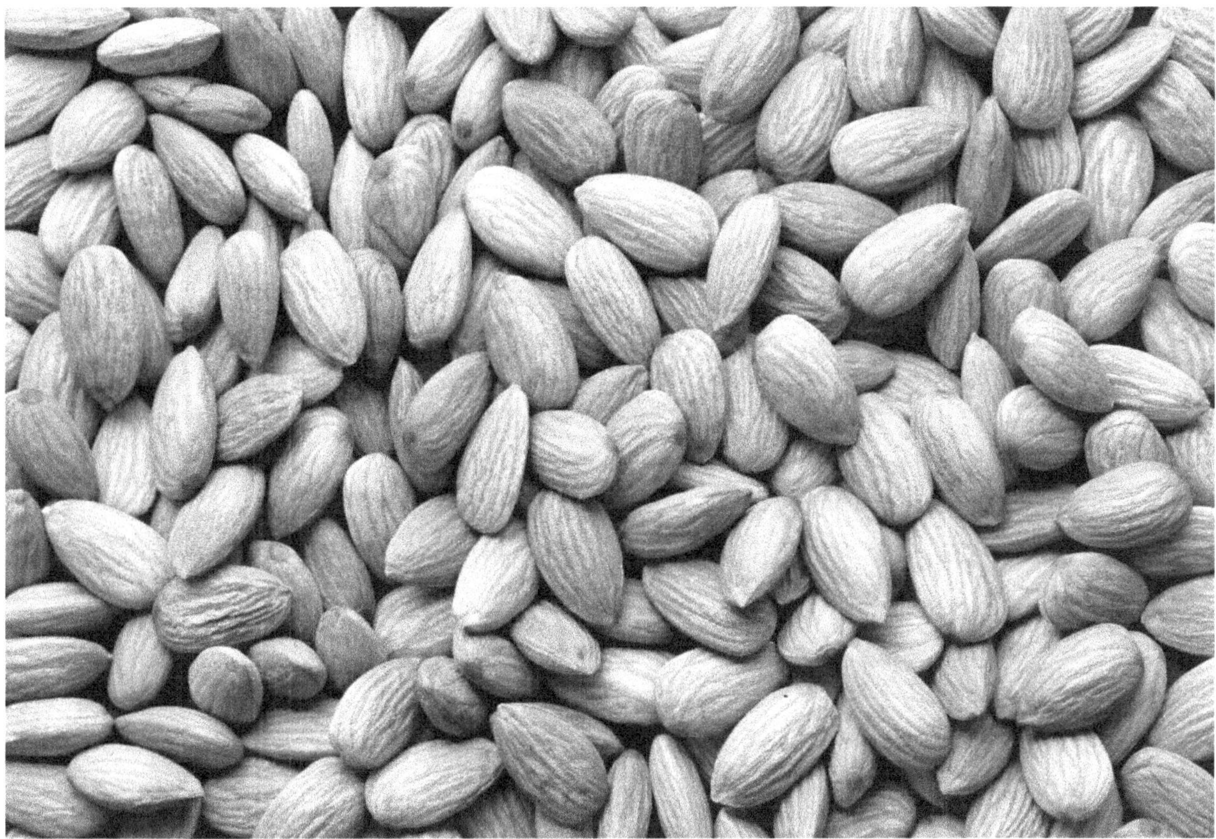

- ○ **Description:** A popular nut known for its crunchy texture and mild flavor.

- ○ **Benefits:** Rich in healthy fats, protein, and fiber, almonds help in maintaining stable blood sugar levels and provide heart-healthy nutrients.

- ○ **Uses:** Snack on raw or roasted almonds, or use almond flour in baking.

- **Chia Seeds:**

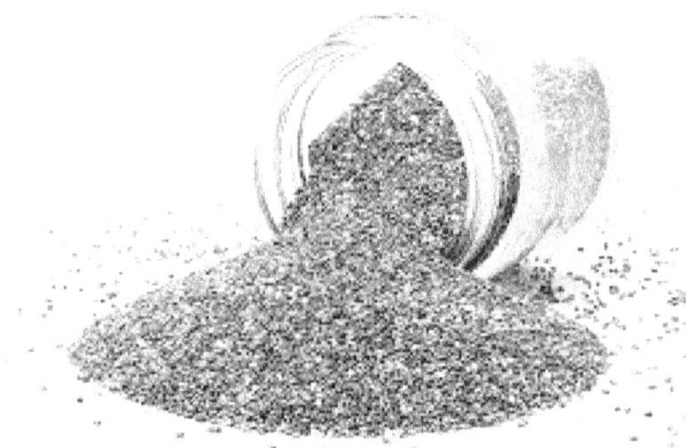

- o **Description:** Tiny seeds with a gelatinous texture when soaked.

- o **Benefits:** Packed with omega-3 fatty acids, fiber, and protein. They help with blood sugar control and are beneficial for heart health.

- o **Uses:** Add to smoothies, make chia pudding, or sprinkle over salads.

- **Flaxseeds:**

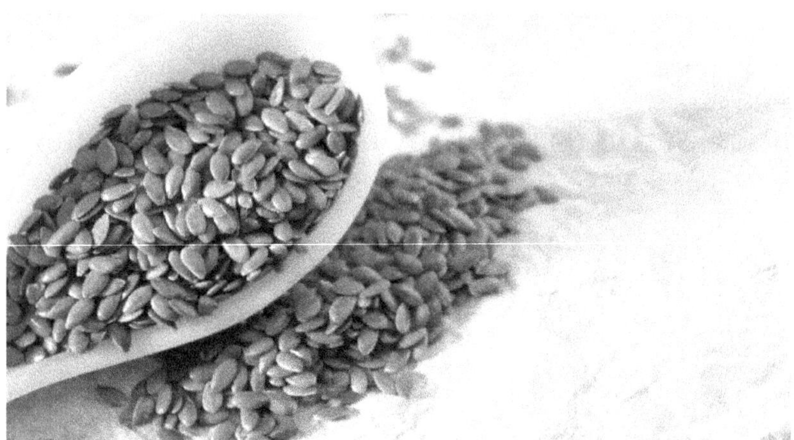

- o **Description:** Small, brown or golden seeds rich in fiber and omega-3 fatty acids.

- o **Benefits:** Support blood sugar regulation and offer cardiovascular benefits.

- o **Uses:** Ground flaxseeds can be added to smoothies, yogurt, or used in baking.

- **Extra Virgin Olive Oil:**

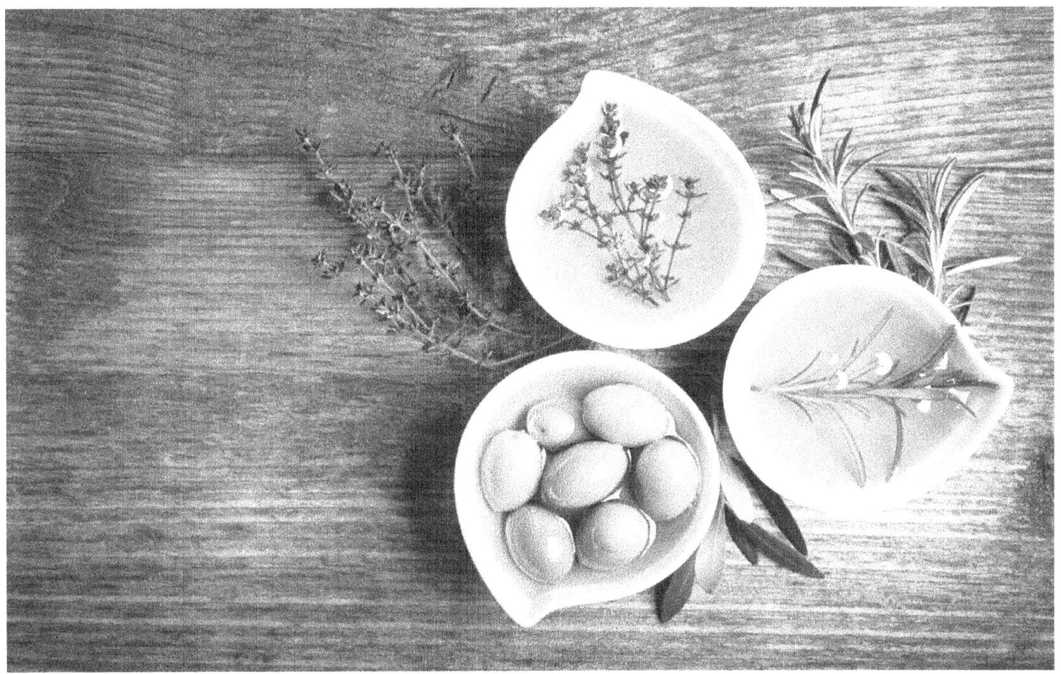

  - o **Description:** Oil obtained from the first cold pressing of olives.

  - o **Benefits:** High in monounsaturated fats and antioxidants, olive oil is beneficial for heart health and has anti-inflammatory properties.

  - o **Uses:** Use for sautéing, dressings, or drizzling over vegetables.

- **Avocado Oil:**

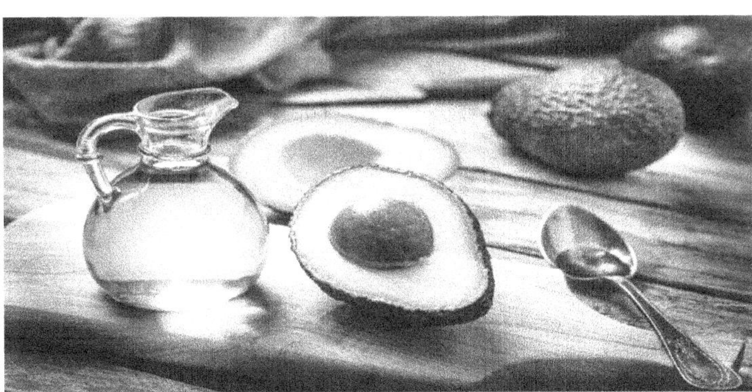

o **Description:** Oil extracted from avocados, known for its high smoke point.

o **Benefits:** Contains monounsaturated fats and vitamin E, which supports heart health and skin health.

o **Uses:** Ideal for high-heat cooking, dressings, or as a finishing oil.

Low-Carb Sweeteners

- **Stevia:**

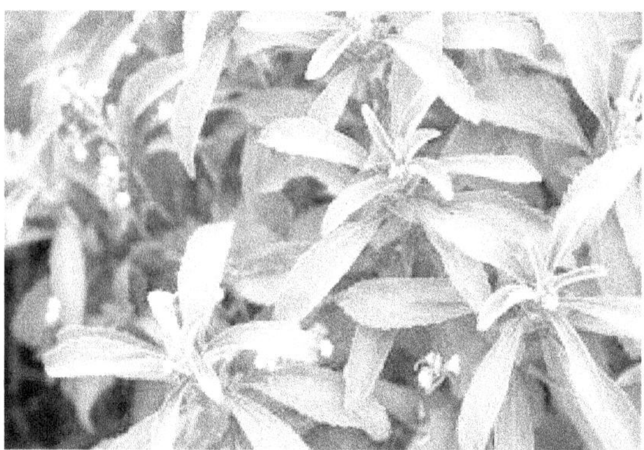

o **Description:** A natural sweetener derived from the leaves of the stevia plant.

o **Benefits:** Zero-calorie and does not affect blood glucose levels.

o **Uses:** Use to sweeten beverages, yogurt, or in baking.

- **Erythritol:**

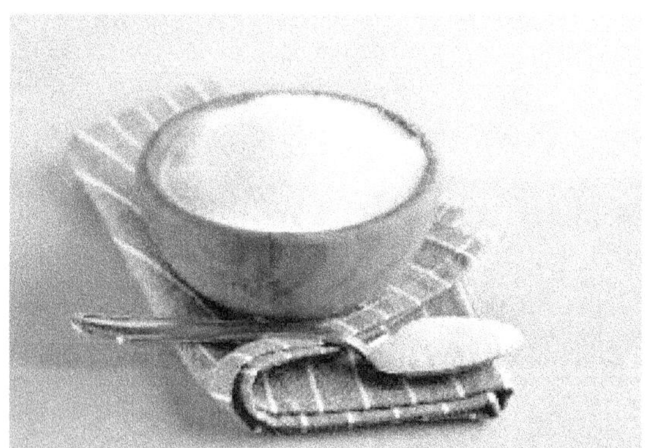

- o **Description:** A sugar alcohol with a mild sweetness.

  - o **Benefits:** Contains almost no calories and has a negligible effect on blood sugar levels.

  - o **Uses:** Ideal for baking, sweetening beverages, or as a sugar substitute in recipes.

- **Monk Fruit Sweetener:**

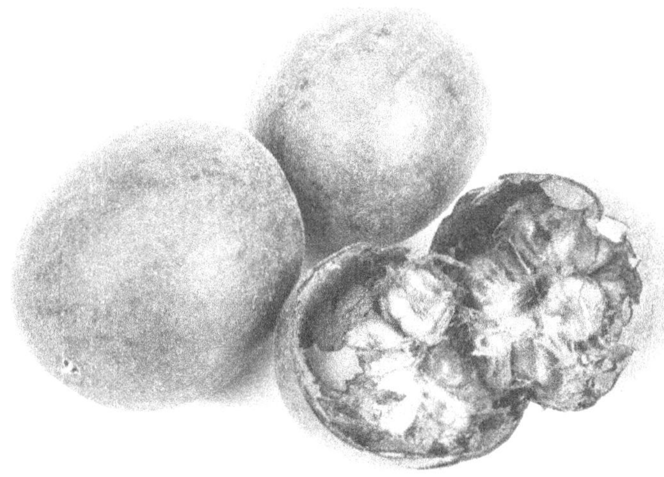

  - o **Description:** A sweetener derived from monk fruit, also known as luo han guo.

  - o **Benefits:** Contains no calories or carbohydrates and does not affect blood sugar.

  - o **Uses:** Use in beverages, baking, and cooking to replace sugar.

Low-Sodium Broths

- **Vegetable Broth:**

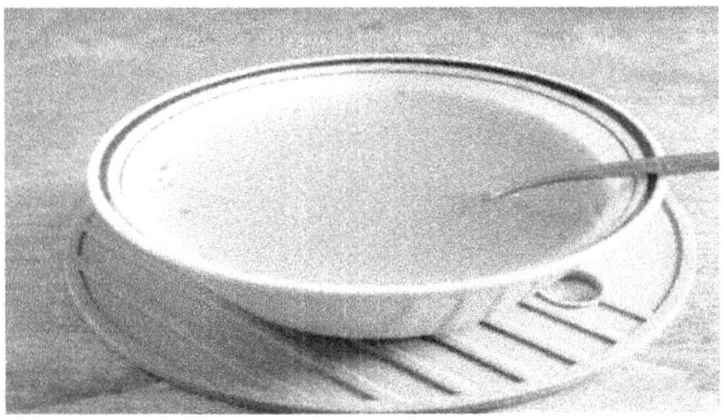

- o **Description:** A liquid made by simmering vegetables and herbs.

- o **Benefits:** Low in sodium and provides a base for soups and stews.

- o **Uses:** Use in soups, sauces, and as a cooking liquid for grains.

- **Chicken Broth:**

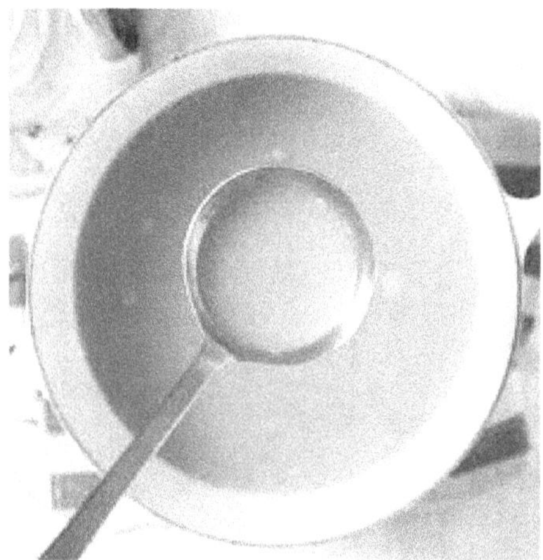

- o **Description:** A liquid made from simmering chicken, vegetables, and herbs.

- o **Benefits:** Choose low-sodium versions to control salt intake while adding flavor.

- o **Uses:** Use for soups, stews, and as a base for cooking.

Spices and Herbs

- **Cinnamon:**

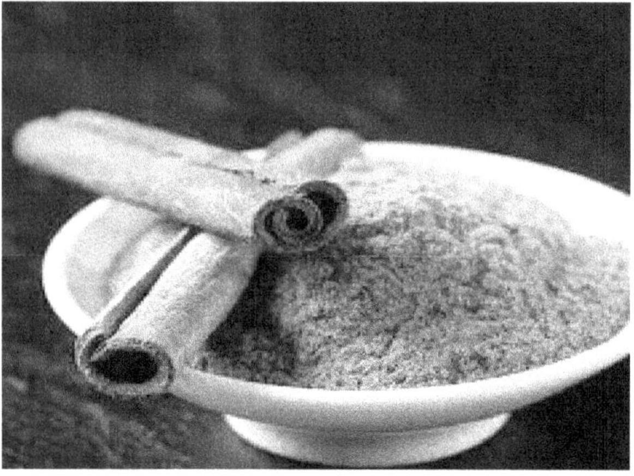

- o **Description:** A spice obtained from the inner bark of trees.

- o **Benefits:** May improve insulin sensitivity and has antioxidant properties.

- o **Uses:** Sprinkle on oatmeal, add to smoothies, or use in baking.

- **Turmeric:**

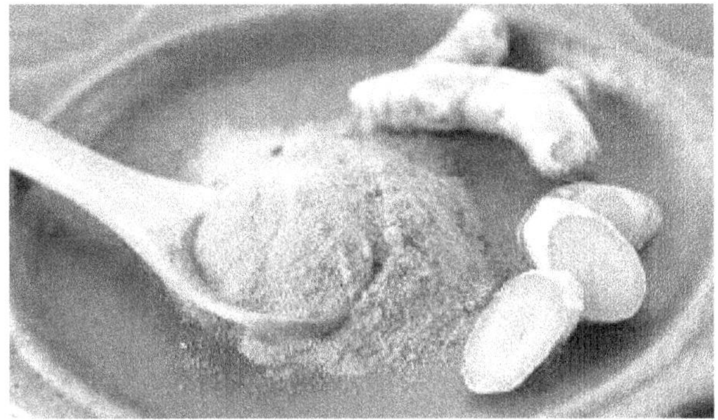

- o **Description:** A bright yellow spice derived from the root of the turmeric plant.

- o **Benefits:** Contains curcumin, which has anti-inflammatory and antioxidant properties.

- o **Uses:** Add to curries, soups, and smoothies for a health boost.

- **Garlic:**

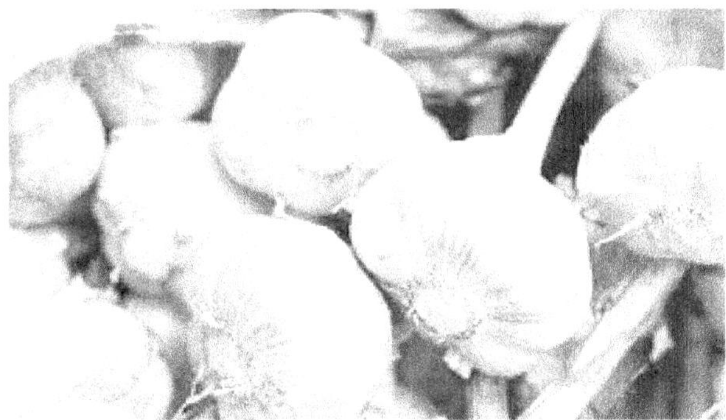

- o **Description:** A pungent herb used for flavoring and medicinal purposes.

- o **Benefits:** Has been shown to have beneficial effects on blood sugar levels and heart health.

- o **Uses:** Incorporate into various dishes, from stir-fries to marinades.

- **Tomatoes:**

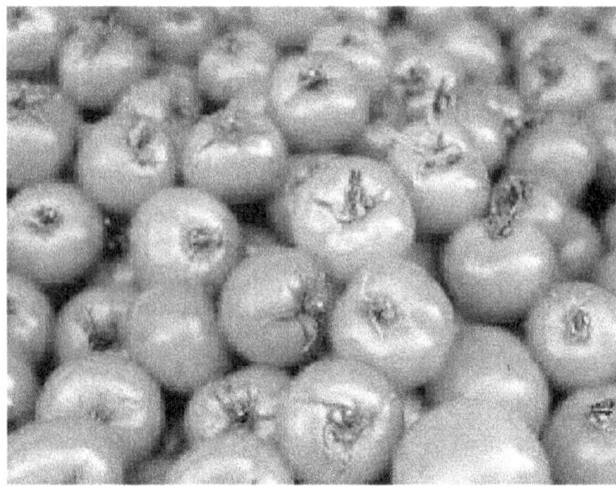

- o **Description:** Available canned, diced, or pureed.

- o **Benefits:** Rich in vitamins and antioxidants like lycopene, which may support heart health.

- o **Uses:** Use in soups, sauces, and stews.

- **Spinach and Kale:**

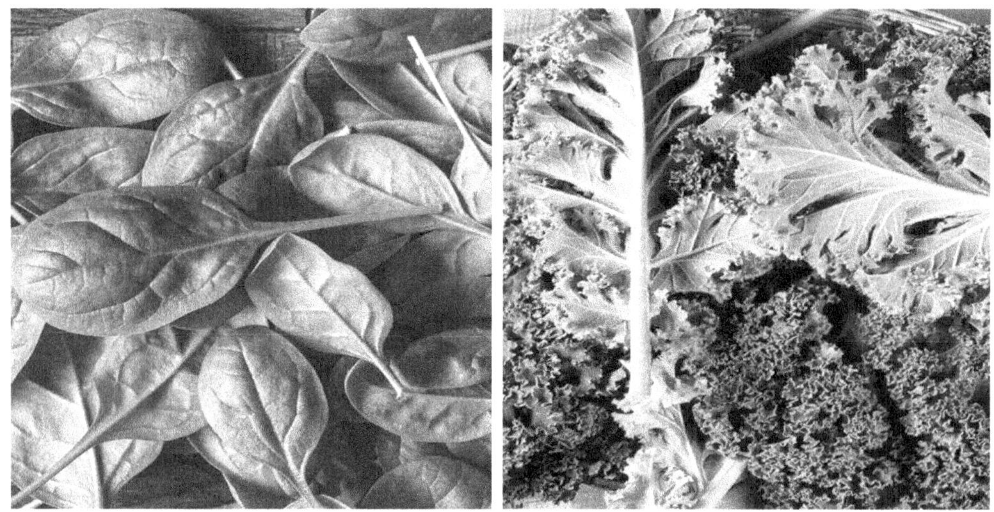

- o **Description:** Leafy greens that are often available frozen.

- o **Benefits:** High in fiber, vitamins, and antioxidants, they support overall health and can aid in blood sugar control.

- o **Uses:** Add to smoothies, soups, and stir-fries.

- **Mustard:**

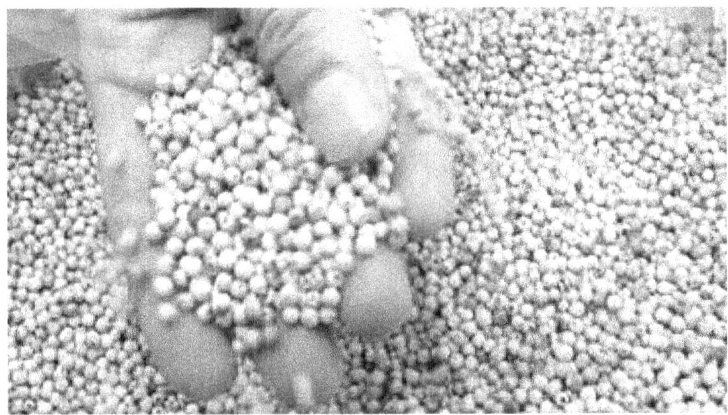

- o **Description:** A tangy condiment made from mustard seeds.

- o **Benefits:** Typically low in sugar and carbs, making it a suitable choice for flavoring.

- o **Uses:** Use as a condiment for meats, in dressings, or as part of marinades.

- **Vinegar:**

- o **Description:** Includes varieties like apple cider vinegar and balsamic vinegar.

- o **Benefits:** May help with blood sugar control and adds flavor without added sugars.

- o **Uses:** Use in salad dressings, marinades, and as a flavor enhancer in cooking.

Kitchen Tools You'll Need

Equipping your kitchen with the right tools is essential for efficient meal preparation and successful management of your dietary needs. Here's a comprehensive list of the must-have kitchen tools:

Cooking Appliances

- **Slow Cooker:**

  - o **Description:** An appliance that cooks food slowly over several hours.

  - o **Benefits:** Allows for hands-off cooking, ideal for making soups, stews, and roasts. It helps in preparing large batches of low-carb meals with minimal effort.

  - o **Uses:** Prepare dishes like chili, beef stew, or pulled chicken.

- **Pressure Cooker/Instant Pot:**

  - o **Description:** A multi-functional appliance that uses high pressure to cook food quickly.

  - o **Benefits:** Reduces cooking time significantly while retaining nutrients and flavors. Great for making soups, stews, and rice.

  - o **Uses:** Cook beans, grains, and tough cuts of meat in a fraction of the time.

- **Air Fryer:**

    o **Description:** An appliance that cooks food using hot air circulation.

    o **Benefits:** Offers a healthier alternative to deep frying by using minimal oil, making it perfect for low-carb snacks and crispy vegetables.

    o **Uses:** Prepare crispy chicken wings, roasted vegetables, or low-carb snacks.

Measuring Tools

- **Digital Kitchen Scale:**

    o **Description:** A scale that provides precise weight measurements for ingredients.

    o **Benefits:** Ensures accuracy in portion sizes and recipe ingredients, essential for managing carb intake.

    o **Uses:** Weigh ingredients for recipes, portion control, and tracking nutritional intake.

- **Measuring Cups and Spoons:**

    o **Description:** Tools for measuring liquid and dry ingredients.

    o **Benefits:** Provides accuracy in ingredient measurements, which is crucial for recipe consistency and nutritional control.

    o **Uses:** Measure ingredients for cooking and baking, ensuring proper proportions.

Prep Tools

- **Chef's Knife:**

- o **Description:** A versatile, sharp knife for general food preparation.

  - o **Benefits:** Allows for efficient chopping, slicing, and dicing of vegetables, fruits, and proteins.

  - o **Uses:** Prepare vegetables, fruits, and meats with ease, making meal prep faster and more efficient.

- **Cutting Boards:**

  - o **Description:** Boards used for cutting and preparing food.

  - o **Benefits:** Prevents cross-contamination and protects countertops. Use separate boards for meats and vegetables.

  - o **Uses:** Chop vegetables, slice meats, and prepare ingredients for cooking.

- **Vegetable Peeler:**

  - o **Description:** A tool for peeling fruits and vegetables.

  - o **Benefits:** Facilitates the removal of skins from vegetables and fruits, which is especially useful for preparing low-carb dishes.

  - o **Uses:** Peel carrots, cucumbers, and other vegetables for salads and cooking.

Cookware

- **Non-Stick Cookware:**

  - o **Description:** Cookware with a coating that prevents food from sticking.

  - o **Benefits:** Requires less oil for cooking, making it easier to prepare low-carb meals with fewer calories.

  - o **Uses:** Cook eggs, pancakes, and stir-fries with minimal oil.

- **Cast Iron Skillet:**

  - o **Description:** A heavy-duty skillet known for even heat distribution.

  - o **Benefits:** Ideal for searing, frying, and baking. It retains heat well and can be used on stovetops and in the oven.

  - o **Uses:** Cook meats, bake cornbread, or prepare frittatas.

- **Baking Sheets:**

  - o **Description:** Flat, rectangular sheets used for baking.

  - o **Benefits:** Ideal for roasting vegetables and baking low-carb treats. Non-stick options make cleanup easier.

  - o **Uses:** Roast vegetables, bake cookies, or make sheet-pan dinners.

Food Storage

- **Glass Containers:**

  - o **Description:** Containers made from glass, often with airtight lids.

  - o **Benefits:** Durable, microwave-safe, and do not retain odors or stains. Great for storing leftovers and prepped ingredients.

  - o **Uses:** Store cooked meals, snacks, and meal prep ingredients.

- **Ziplock Bags:**

  - o **Description:** Reusable plastic bags with a sealing mechanism.

  - o **Benefits:** Convenient for portioning and freezing foods, ensuring freshness and easy access.

  - o **Uses:** Store frozen fruits, prepped vegetables, and portioned meats.

- **Spatula:**

    - **Description:** A tool for stirring, flipping, and serving food.

    - **Benefits:** Silicone or wooden spatulas are gentle on non-stick cookware and help prevent scratching.

    - **Uses:** Stir sauces, flip pancakes, and serve dishes.

- **Tongs:**

    - **Description:** A tool used for gripping and turning food.

    - **Benefits:** Allows for easy handling of hot or delicate items without direct contact.

    - **Uses:** Turn meats on the grill, toss salads, or serve pasta.

- **Whisk:**

    - **Description:** A tool used for mixing and blending ingredients.

    - **Benefits:** Ideal for incorporating air into mixtures, such as beating eggs or whipping cream.

    - **Uses:** Mix dressings, beat eggs, and combine dry ingredients.

Miscellaneous Tools

- **Food Processor:**

    - **Description:** An appliance that processes food through various attachments.

    - **Benefits:** Versatile for chopping, slicing, shredding, and blending, which speeds up meal preparation.

    - **Uses:** Make sauces, chop vegetables, and prepare dough.

- **Blender:**

    - ○ **Description:** An appliance used to blend and puree ingredients.

    - ○ **Benefits:** Essential for making smoothies, soups, and sauces. Helps achieve a smooth consistency in recipes.

    - ○ **Uses:** Blend fruits and vegetables, make smoothies, and prepare soups.

By incorporating these essential ingredients and tools into your kitchen, you'll be well-equipped to prepare a variety of delicious, diabetic-friendly meals that support your health and well-being. These staples and tools not only simplify meal preparation but also ensure that you can manage your dietary needs effectively.

This detailed guide provides an extensive look at pantry staples and kitchen tools, ensuring you have all the necessary components to create a successful and healthy diabetic meal plan.

CHAPTER 2

BREAKFAST RECIPES

Breakfast is a crucial meal, especially for those managing diabetes. It's an opportunity to set the tone for stable blood sugar levels throughout the day and ensure sustained energy. This selection of breakfast recipes focuses on low-carb and low-sugar options that are not only nutritious but also varied and satisfying. Each recipe is crafted to meet dietary needs while providing delicious, filling options to start your day right.

1. Avocado and Egg Breakfast Bowl

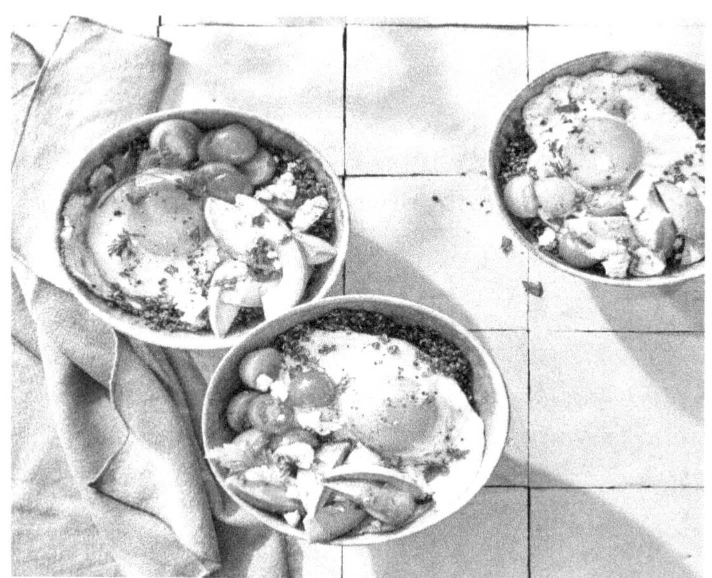

Description: This Avocado and Egg Breakfast Bowl combines the creamy, rich texture of avocado with the high-quality protein of eggs. It's a quick and versatile meal that provides a hearty start to your day.

Ingredients:

- 1 ripe avocado

- 2 large eggs

- 1 tablespoon olive oil

- Salt and pepper to taste

- Optional toppings: cherry tomatoes, red pepper flakes, fresh herbs (such as cilantro or chives), a squeeze of lemon juice

Instructions:

1. **Prepare Avocado:** Cut the avocado in half and remove the pit. Scoop the flesh into a bowl, lightly mash if preferred, and season with a pinch of salt and a squeeze of lemon juice to taste.

2. **Cook Eggs:** Heat olive oil in a non-stick skillet over medium heat. Crack the eggs into the pan and cook until the whites are set and the yolks are cooked to your preference (sunny-side up, poached, or scrambled).

3. **Assemble Bowl:** Place the cooked eggs on top of the avocado. Season with additional salt, pepper, and any optional toppings you like.

4. **Serve:** Enjoy immediately while the eggs are warm.

Why It's Great: This dish is packed with healthy fats from avocado and protein from eggs. It helps keep you full longer and maintains stable blood sugar levels, making it ideal for a diabetic-friendly breakfast.

2. Greek Yogurt with Berries and Nuts

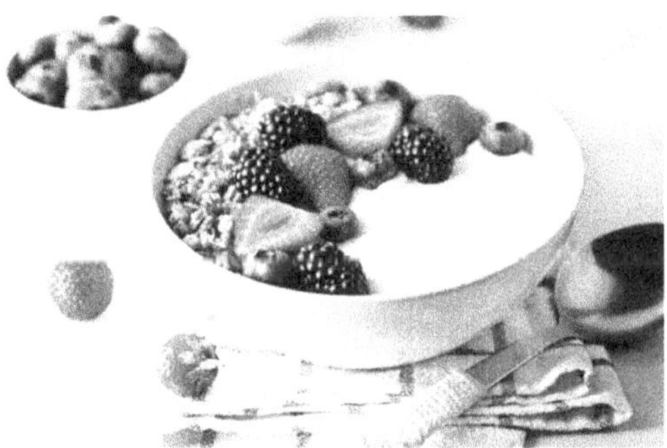

Description: Greek Yogurt with Berries and Nuts is a simple yet nutrient-dense breakfast option. It combines creamy Greek yogurt with the freshness of berries and the crunch of nuts, offering a balanced mix of protein, fiber, and antioxidants.

Ingredients:

- 1 cup plain Greek yogurt (unsweetened)

- 1/2 cup mixed fresh berries (blueberries, strawberries, raspberries)

- 2 tablespoons chopped nuts (almonds, walnuts, or pecans)

- 1 teaspoon chia seeds (optional)

- 1 tablespoon honey or a low-carb sweetener (optional)

Instructions:

1. **Prepare Yogurt:** Spoon the Greek yogurt into a bowl.

2. **Add Toppings:** Top with mixed berries and chopped nuts. Sprinkle chia seeds over the top if using.

3. **Sweeten (Optional):** Drizzle with honey or a low-carb sweetener if desired.

4. **Serve:** Enjoy immediately or cover and refrigerate for a quick grab-and-go breakfast.

Why It's Great: Greek yogurt provides a high protein content, while berries add fiber and antioxidants. Nuts contribute healthy fats, making this breakfast both satisfying and beneficial for managing blood sugar levels.

3. Low Carb Chia Seed Pudding

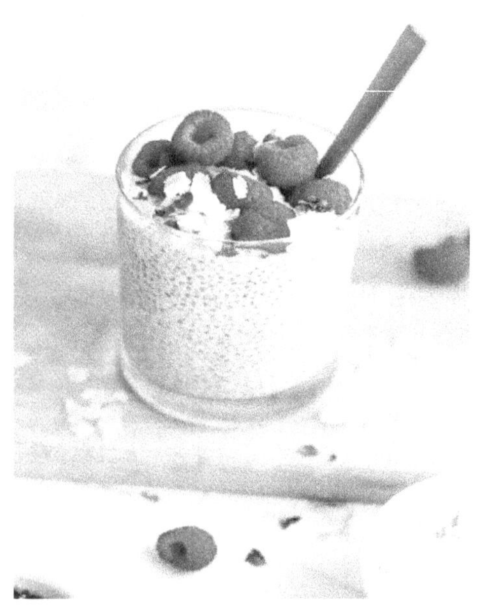

Description: Low Carb Chia Seed Pudding is a versatile and filling breakfast that can be prepared in advance. It's rich in fiber and omega-3 fatty acids, which are beneficial for overall health and diabetes management.

Ingredients:

- 3 tablespoons chia seeds

- 1 cup unsweetened almond milk (or any

low-carb milk alternative)

- 1 teaspoon vanilla extract

- Sweetener of choice (stevia, erythritol, or monk fruit) to taste

- Optional toppings: fresh berries, sliced almonds, coconut flakes, a dollop of Greek yogurt

Instructions:

1. **Mix Ingredients:** In a bowl, combine chia seeds, almond milk, vanilla extract, and sweetener. Stir well to ensure the chia seeds are fully mixed.

2. **Refrigerate:** Cover and refrigerate for at least 4 hours or overnight until the mixture thickens into a pudding-like consistency.

3. **Add Toppings:** Before serving, add your choice of toppings to enhance flavor and texture.

4. **Serve:** Enjoy chilled.

Why It's Great: Chia seeds are a great source of fiber and healthy fats, which aid in blood sugar control and promote satiety. This pudding is also easy to customize with various toppings.

4. Almond Flour Pancakes

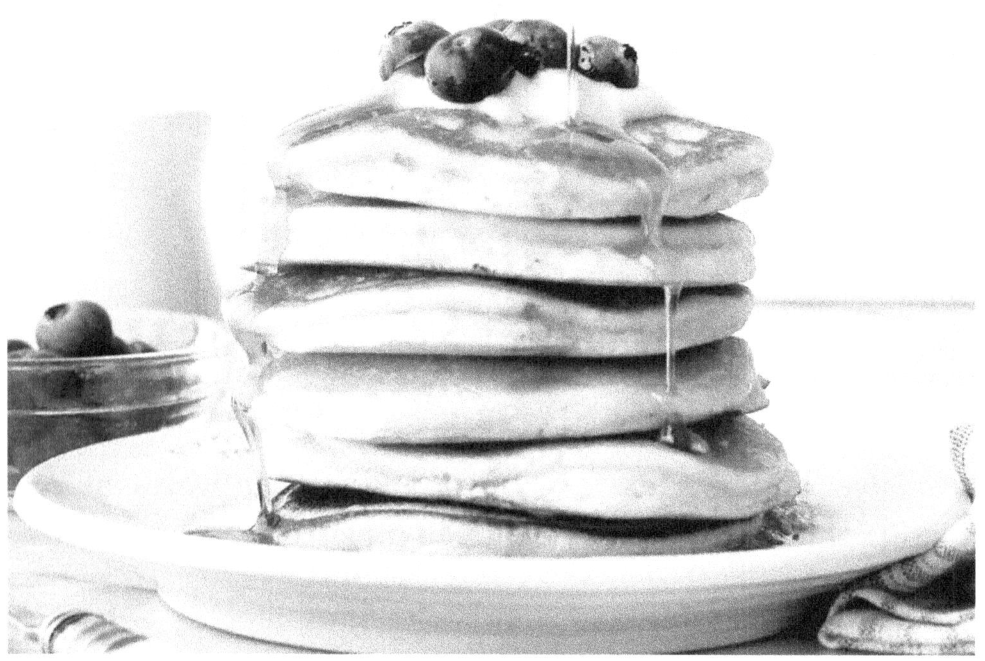

Description: Almond Flour Pancakes are a delicious, low-carb alternative to traditional pancakes. They're perfect for a hearty breakfast that won't spike blood sugar levels.

Ingredients:

- 1 cup almond flour

- 2 large eggs

- 1/4 cup unsweetened almond milk

- 1/4 cup melted coconut oil or butter

- 1 tablespoon honey or a low-carb sweetener

- 1 teaspoon baking powder

- 1/2 teaspoon vanilla extract

- Butter or oil for cooking

Instructions:

1. **Prepare Batter:** In a bowl, mix almond flour, eggs, almond milk, melted coconut oil, honey, baking powder, and vanilla extract until smooth.

2. **Cook Pancakes:** Heat a skillet over medium heat and add a little butter or oil. Pour batter onto the skillet to form pancakes. Cook until bubbles form on the surface, then flip and cook until golden brown on both sides.

3. **Serve:** Serve warm with fresh berries, sugar-free syrup, or a dollop of Greek yogurt.

Why It's Great: Almond flour is low in carbs and high in protein and healthy fats, making these pancakes a filling and diabetes-friendly option. They also offer a good amount of fiber and essential nutrients.

5. Spinach and Feta Omelette

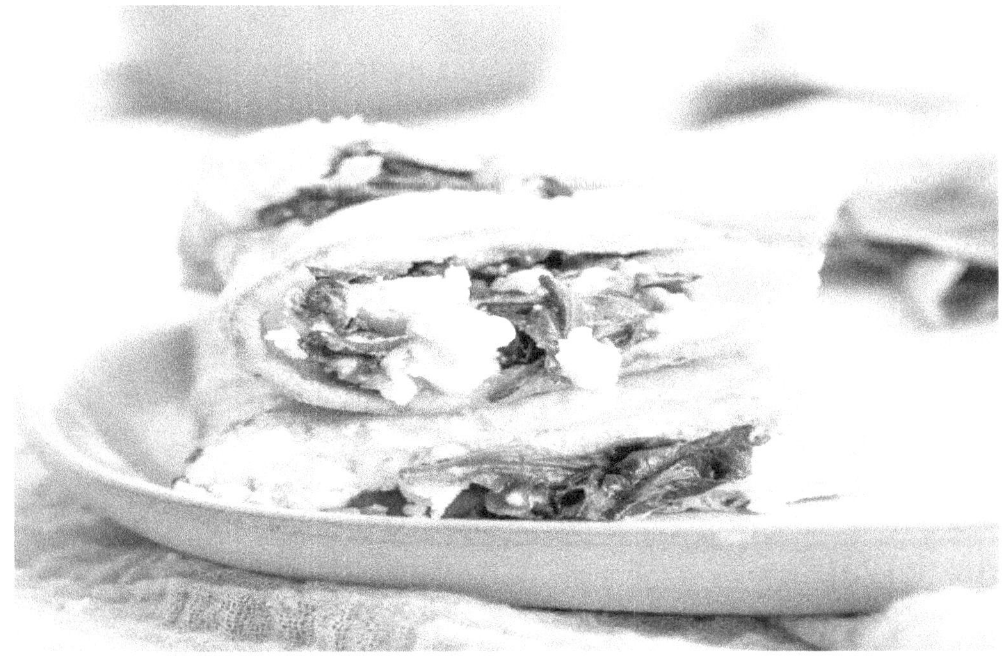

Description: Spinach and Feta Omelette is a savory breakfast that provides a satisfying mix of protein and vegetables. It's easy to make and offers a flavorful way to include more greens in your diet.

Ingredients:

- 3 large eggs

- 1 cup fresh spinach, chopped

- 1/4 cup feta cheese, crumbled

- 1 tablespoon olive oil or butter

- Salt and pepper to taste

- Optional: diced tomatoes, onions, bell peppers

Instructions:

1. **Prepare Filling:** Heat olive oil or butter in a non-stick skillet over medium heat. Add spinach and cook until wilted.

2. **Cook Omelette:** In a bowl, whisk eggs with salt and pepper. Pour eggs into the skillet over the spinach. Cook until edges start to set. Sprinkle feta cheese (and any optional ingredients) on one half of the omelette.

3. **Fold and Serve:** Fold the omelette in half and cook until fully set. Serve warm.

Why It's Great: Spinach is rich in vitamins and minerals, while feta cheese adds a creamy texture and protein. This omelette is both nutritious and filling, supporting stable blood sugar levels.

6. Coconut Flour Waffles

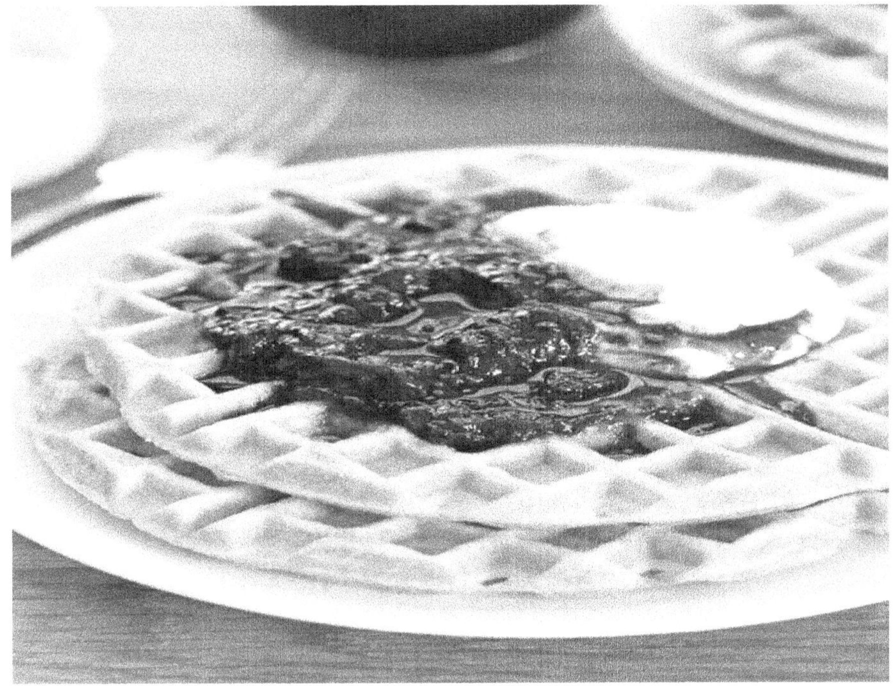

Description: Coconut Flour Waffles are a delightful low-carb option that can be enjoyed with various toppings. They're perfect for a weekend breakfast or brunch.

Ingredients:

- 1/2 cup coconut flour

- 4 large eggs

- 1/4 cup unsweetened almond milk

- 1/4 cup melted coconut oil

- 1 tablespoon honey or a low-carb sweetener

- 1 teaspoon baking powder

- Pinch of salt

Instructions:

1. **Prepare Batter:** In a bowl, mix coconut flour, eggs, almond milk, melted coconut oil, honey, baking powder, and salt until smooth.

2. **Cook Waffles:** Pour batter into a preheated waffle iron and cook according to the manufacturer's instructions until golden brown.

3. **Serve:** Top with fresh berries, a dollop of Greek yogurt, or a sprinkle of cinnamon.

Why It's Great: Coconut flour is low in carbs and high in fiber, making these waffles a good choice for managing blood sugar levels while providing a satisfying meal.

7. Breakfast Smoothie with Spinach and Protein Powder

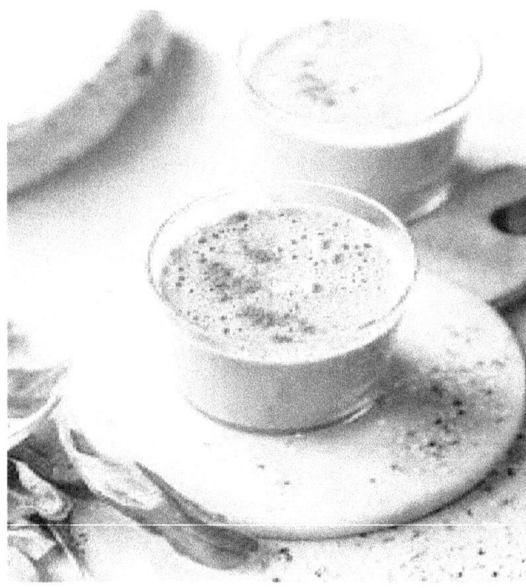

Description: This Breakfast Smoothie with Spinach and Protein Powder is a quick, nutrient-packed option that's perfect for busy mornings.

Ingredients:

- 1 cup unsweetened almond milk

- 1 scoop protein powder (vanilla or unflavored)

- 1 cup fresh spinach

- 1/2 banana

- 1 tablespoon flaxseeds or chia seeds

- Ice cubes (optional)

- Optional: a few drops of vanilla extract or a small handful of frozen berries

Instructions:

1. **Blend Ingredients:** Combine almond milk, protein powder, spinach, banana, and flaxseeds in a blender. Blend until smooth.

2. **Adjust Consistency:** Add ice cubes if desired for a thicker texture or a few drops of vanilla extract for extra flavor.

3. **Serve:** Pour into a glass and enjoy.

Why It's Great: This smoothie provides a balanced mix of protein, fiber, and vitamins. Spinach adds essential nutrients without affecting the flavor, making it a great option for a healthy, quick breakfast.

8. Cottage Cheese with Fresh Berries

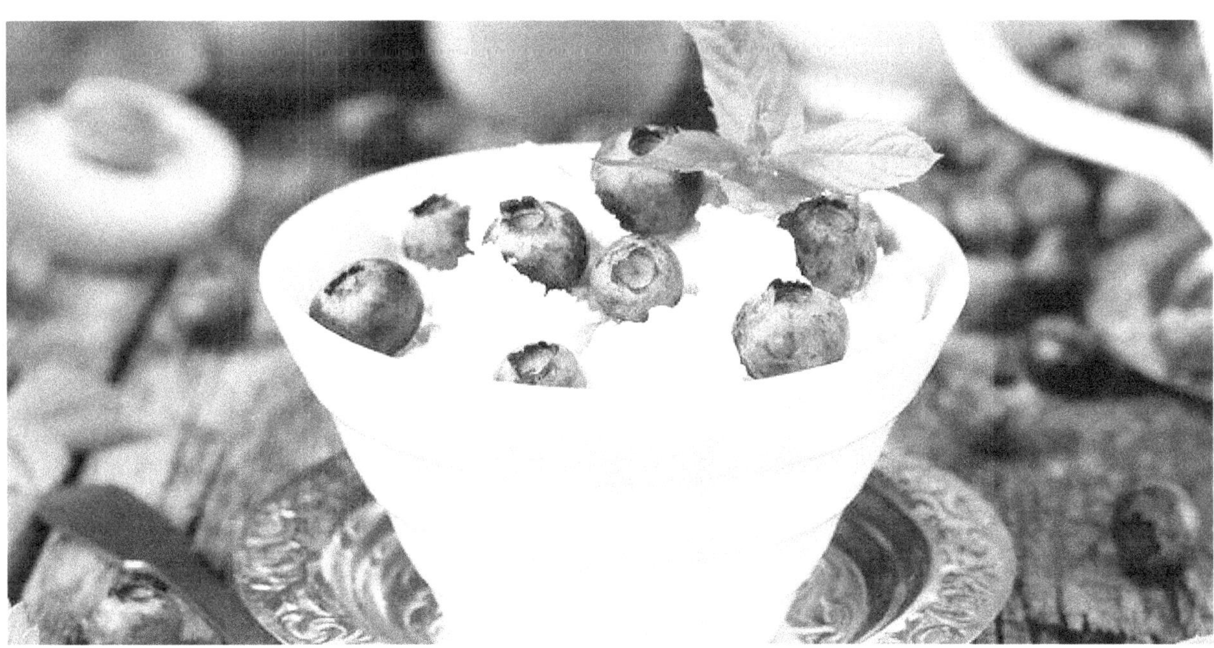

Description: Cottage Cheese with Fresh Berries is a light yet nutritious breakfast that combines protein-rich cottage cheese with the sweet, tangy flavor of berries.

Ingredients:

- 1 cup low-fat cottage cheese

- 1/2 cup mixed fresh berries (strawberries, blueberries, raspberries)

- 1 tablespoon chopped nuts (optional, such as almonds or walnuts)

- 1 teaspoon honey or a low-carb sweetener (optional)

Instructions:

1. **Assemble Bowl:** Scoop cottage cheese into a bowl and top with fresh berries.

2. **Add Toppings:** Sprinkle with chopped nuts and a drizzle of honey if desired.

3. **Serve:** Enjoy immediately or refrigerate for a quick grab-and-go option.

Why It's Great: Cottage cheese is high in protein and low in carbs, while berries provide antioxidants and fiber. This breakfast is both satisfying and beneficial for managing blood sugar.

9. Low Carb Breakfast Burrito with Turkey Sausage

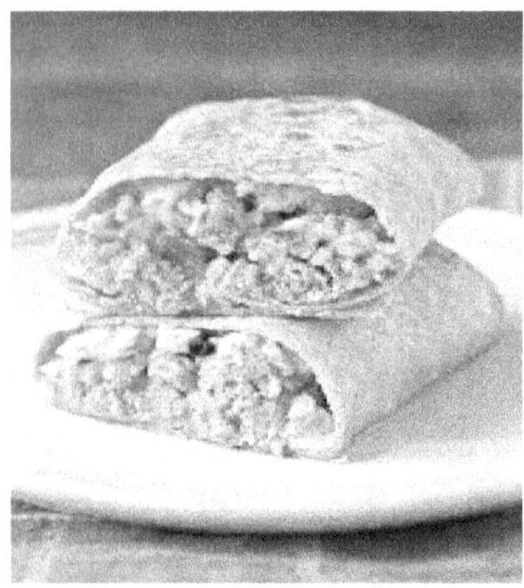

Description: The Low Carb Breakfast Burrito with Turkey Sausage is a savory option that's perfect for those who enjoy a hearty breakfast wrap without the carbs.

Ingredients:

- 1 low-carb tortilla or wrap

- 2 turkey sausage links, cooked and crumbled

- 1 large egg

- 1/4 cup shredded cheddar cheese

- 1/4 cup diced bell peppers

- 1/4 cup chopped onions

- 1 tablespoon olive oil

- Salsa or hot sauce (optional)

Instructions:

1. **Cook Vegetables:** Heat olive oil in a skillet and sauté bell peppers and onions until tender.

2. **Prepare Egg:** Scramble the egg and add it to the skillet with the vegetables. Cook until fully set.

3. **Assemble Burrito:** Place the turkey sausage, egg mixture, and cheese in the low-carb tortilla. Roll up tightly.

4. **Serve:** Enjoy with a side of salsa or hot sauce if desired.

Why It's Great: This burrito is rich in protein and low in carbs, making it a filling and diabetes-friendly breakfast option that provides sustained energy.

10. Smoked Salmon and Avocado Toast on Low Carb Bread

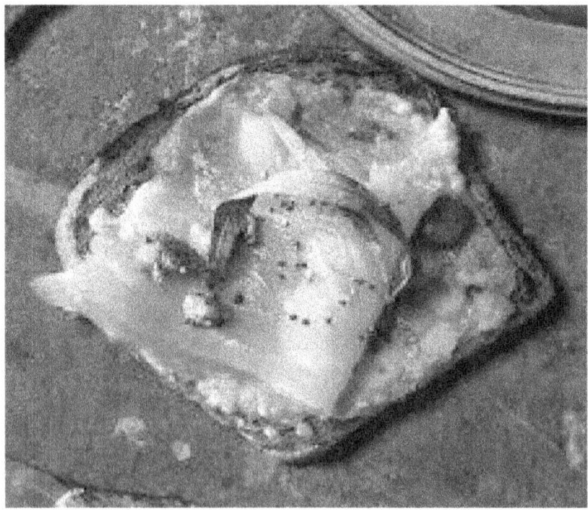

Description: Smoked Salmon and Avocado Toast on Low Carb Bread is a sophisticated yet simple breakfast that combines the rich flavors of smoked salmon with creamy avocado on a low-carb base.

Ingredients:

- 1 slice low-carb bread

- 1/2 avocado

- 2 ounces smoked salmon

- 1 tablespoon cream cheese (optional)

- Lemon juice

- Salt and pepper to taste

- Capers or fresh dill for garnish (optional)

Instructions:

1. **Prepare Toast:** Toast the low-carb bread until crispy.

2. **Mash Avocado:** Mash the avocado and spread it over the toasted bread. Season with a squeeze of lemon juice, salt, and pepper.

3. **Add Toppings:** Place smoked salmon on top of the avocado spread. Add a thin layer of cream cheese if using.

4. **Garnish:** Top with capers or fresh dill if desired.

Why It's Great: This breakfast offers a perfect balance of healthy fats from avocado and salmon, along with the low-carb base of the bread, making it both satisfying and suitable for blood sugar control.

Each of these recipes has been crafted to ensure that you have a variety of breakfast options that are not only low in carbs and sugar but also full of flavor and nutrients. Enjoy exploring these recipes and finding your favorites to kickstart your day with a healthy and enjoyable breakfast.

CHAPTER 3

LUNCH RECIPES

Lunch is a vital meal, especially for those managing diabetes. It should provide enough energy to keep you going through the afternoon while maintaining stable blood sugar levels. These lunch recipes are designed with that in mind, offering a variety of flavors, textures, and nutrients. Each recipe is low in carbohydrates and sugar, making them perfect choices for those who need to manage their blood sugar carefully. Let's dive into these delicious and healthy lunch options.

1. Grilled Chicken Salad with Avocado

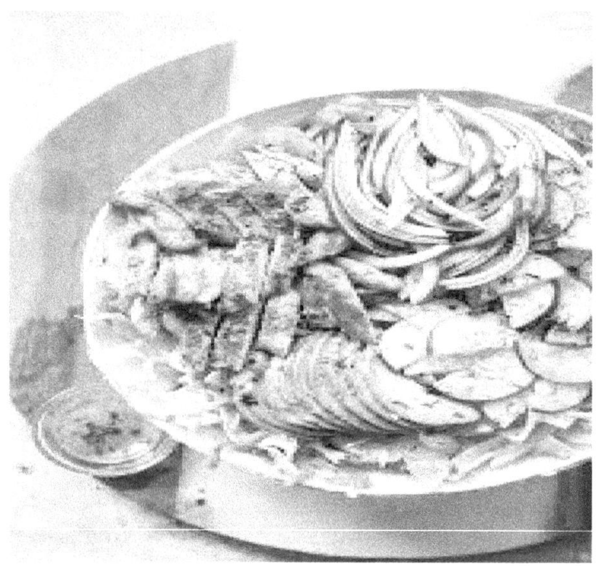

Description: Grilled Chicken Salad with Avocado is a classic, yet satisfying lunch option that combines lean protein with healthy fats and fiber. This salad is not only filling but also packed with nutrients that support overall health, particularly for those with diabetes.

Ingredients:

- 2 grilled chicken breasts, sliced

- 1 ripe avocado, diced

- 4 cups mixed salad greens (such as spinach, arugula, and romaine)

- 1/2 cup cherry tomatoes, halved

- 1/4 cup red onion, thinly sliced

- 1/4 cup cucumber, sliced

- 1/4 cup crumbled feta cheese (optional)

- 2 tablespoons olive oil

- 1 tablespoon balsamic vinegar

- Salt and pepper to taste

Instructions:

1. **Prepare Ingredients:** Grill the chicken breasts and slice them once cooled. Dice the avocado and prepare the other vegetables.

2. **Assemble Salad:** In a large bowl, combine salad greens, tomatoes, red onion, cucumber, and avocado. Top with sliced chicken and crumbled feta cheese if using.

3. **Dress Salad:** Drizzle with olive oil and balsamic vinegar. Season with salt and pepper to taste.

4. **Serve:** Toss the salad lightly and serve immediately.

Why It's Great: This salad is rich in protein and healthy fats, making it a balanced and diabetes-friendly meal. The avocado provides monounsaturated fats, which are beneficial for heart health, while the chicken offers lean protein to help keep you full longer.

2. Zucchini Noodles with Pesto and Grilled Shrimp

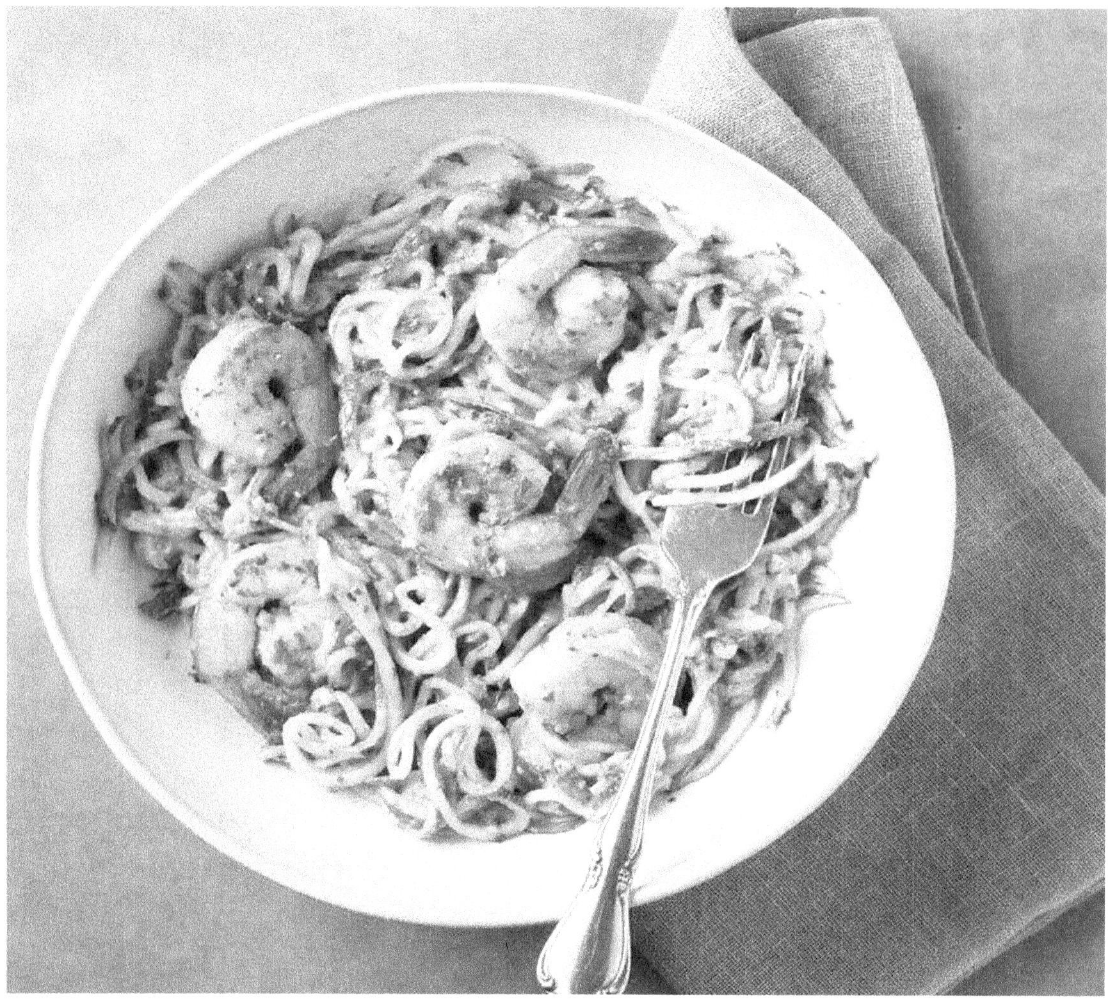

Description: Zucchini Noodles with Pesto and Grilled Shrimp is a light, yet flavorful dish that's perfect for lunch. This low-carb alternative to traditional pasta offers the same satisfaction but with fewer calories and carbs, making it ideal for blood sugar control.

Ingredients:

- 2 medium zucchinis, spiralized into noodles

- 12 large shrimp, peeled and deveined

- 2 tablespoons olive oil

- 1/2 cup fresh basil pesto (store-bought or homemade)

- 1/4 cup cherry tomatoes, halved

- Salt and pepper to taste

- Optional garnish: freshly grated Parmesan cheese and pine nuts

Instructions:

1. **Grill Shrimp:** Heat 1 tablespoon of olive oil in a grill pan over medium heat. Season shrimp with salt and pepper, then grill until pink and opaque, about 2-3 minutes per side.

2. **Cook Zucchini Noodles:** In a separate pan, heat the remaining olive oil over medium heat. Add zucchini noodles and sauté for 2-3 minutes until slightly tender.

3. **Combine and Serve:** Toss the zucchini noodles with pesto and cherry tomatoes. Add the grilled shrimp on top and garnish with Parmesan cheese and pine nuts if desired.

Why It's Great: Zucchini noodles are a fantastic low-carb alternative to pasta, and they pair wonderfully with the rich flavors of pesto and shrimp. This dish is light yet satisfying, making it a perfect lunch option for those managing diabetes.

3. Low Carb Chicken Caesar Wrap

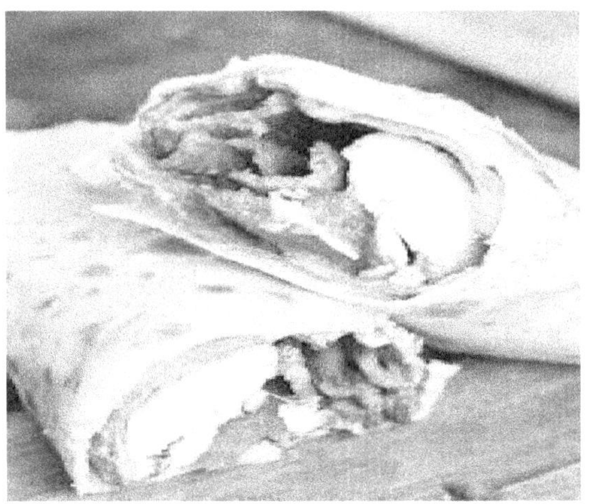

Description: The Low Carb Chicken Caesar Wrap is a portable and convenient lunch option that combines all the flavors of a classic Caesar salad in a wrap. It's perfect for on-the-go meals and provides a balanced mix of protein and healthy fats.

Ingredients:

- 1 large low-carb tortilla or wrap

- 1 grilled chicken breast, sliced

- 2 cups romaine lettuce, chopped

- 1/4 cup grated Parmesan cheese

- 2 tablespoons Caesar dressing (low-carb or homemade)

- Optional: a few slices of avocado or bacon bits for extra flavor

Instructions:

1. **Prepare Ingredients:** Grill the chicken and slice it into strips. Chop the lettuce.

2. **Assemble Wrap:** Lay the tortilla flat and layer with lettuce, chicken, Parmesan cheese, and Caesar dressing. Add avocado or bacon if desired.

3. **Wrap and Serve:** Roll up the tortilla tightly, slice in half, and serve immediately.

Why It's Great: This wrap is low in carbs and high in protein, making it a satisfying and diabetes-friendly lunch option. The Caesar dressing adds creaminess and flavor, while the chicken provides lean protein to keep you full.

4. Mediterranean Tuna Salad

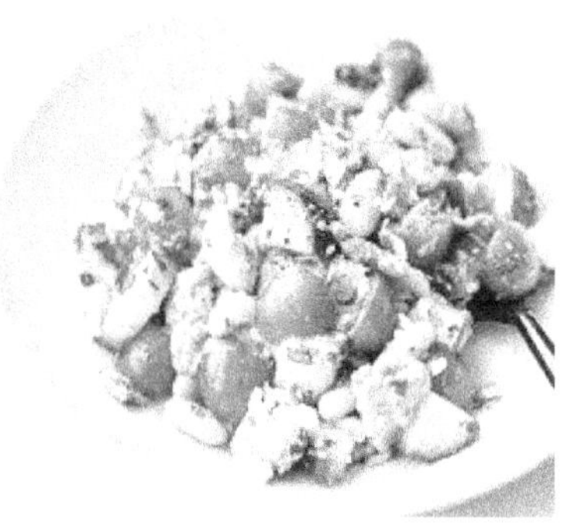

Description: Mediterranean Tuna Salad is a flavorful and nutrient-packed dish that's both refreshing and satisfying. This salad is rich in omega-3 fatty acids, which are beneficial for heart health, and it's also low in carbs, making it an excellent choice for managing blood sugar levels.

Ingredients:

- 1 can of tuna in olive oil, drained
- 1/2 cup cherry tomatoes, halved
- 1/4 cup cucumber, diced
- 1/4 cup red onion, finely chopped
- 1/4 cup Kalamata olives, pitted and sliced
- 2 tablespoons capers, rinsed
- 2 tablespoons olive oil
- 1 tablespoon red wine vinegar
- 1 teaspoon dried oregano
- Salt and pepper to taste
- Optional: 1/4 cup crumbled feta cheese

Instructions:

1. **Prepare Salad:** In a large bowl, combine tuna, cherry tomatoes, cucumber, red onion, olives, and capers.
2. **Dress Salad:** Drizzle with olive oil and red wine vinegar. Add dried oregano, salt, and pepper to taste. Toss well to combine.
3. **Serve:** Serve chilled, with or without a sprinkle of feta cheese.

Why It's Great: This salad is packed with flavor and nutrients, thanks to the combination of fresh vegetables, tuna, and olives. It's also rich in healthy fats and low in carbs, making it perfect for a diabetes-friendly lunch.

5. Spinach and Mushroom Stuffed Chicken Breast

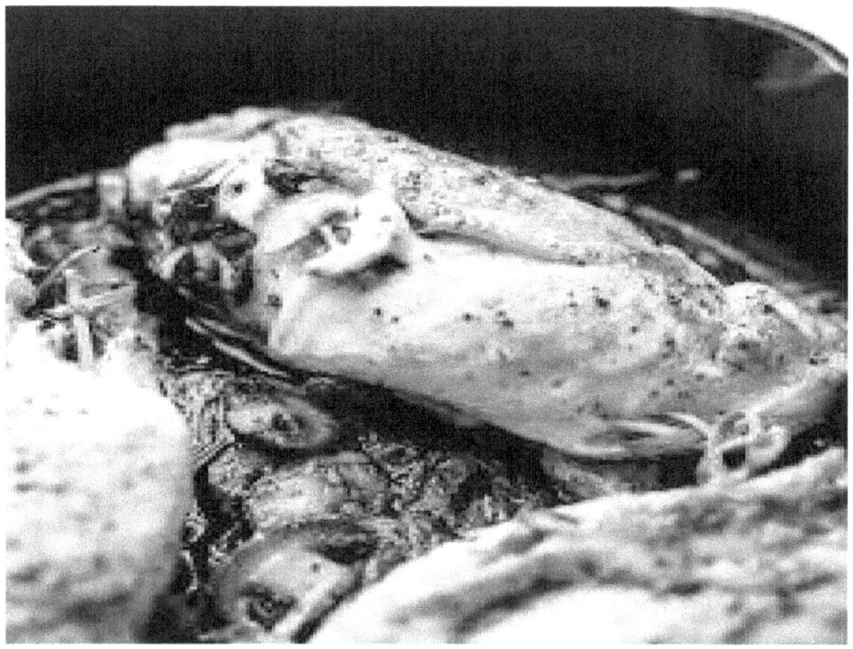

Description: Spinach and Mushroom Stuffed Chicken Breast is a flavorful, protein-rich dish that makes a hearty lunch. The stuffing of spinach and mushrooms adds moisture and a burst of flavor, while the chicken provides a lean protein source.

Ingredients:

- 2 large chicken breasts, butterflied

- 1 cup fresh spinach, chopped

- 1/2 cup mushrooms, finely chopped

- 1/4 cup ricotta or cream cheese

- 2 tablespoons grated Parmesan cheese

- 2 cloves garlic, minced

- 1 tablespoon olive oil

- Salt and pepper to taste

Instructions:

1. **Prepare Filling:** Heat olive oil in a skillet over medium heat. Sauté garlic, spinach, and mushrooms until soft. Remove from heat and stir in ricotta or cream cheese and Parmesan. Season with salt and pepper.

2. **Stuff Chicken:** Open the butterflied chicken breasts and fill them with the spinach and mushroom mixture. Fold the chicken over and secure with toothpicks.

3. **Cook Chicken:** In the same skillet, add a bit more olive oil and cook the stuffed chicken breasts over medium heat until golden brown and fully cooked, about 5-7 minutes per side.

4. **Serve:** Slice and serve with a side of steamed vegetables or a small salad.

Why It's Great: This dish is rich in protein and packed with nutrients from the spinach and mushrooms. It's also low in carbs, making it a satisfying and diabetes-friendly lunch option.

6. Turkey Lettuce Wraps

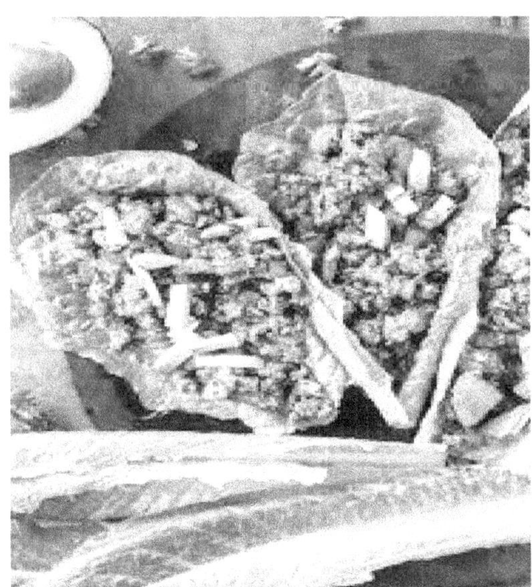

Description: Turkey Lettuce Wraps are a light and refreshing lunch option that's easy to make and perfect for those looking to cut down on carbs. These wraps are versatile and can be filled with a variety of flavors, making them a great go-to for a quick and healthy lunch.

Ingredients:

- 8 large lettuce leaves (such as romaine or butter lettuce)

- 1/2 pound ground turkey

- 1/4 cup onions, diced

- 1/4 cup bell peppers, diced

- 2 cloves garlic, minced

- 1 tablespoon soy sauce or tamari

- 1 teaspoon sesame oil

- 1/2 teaspoon ground ginger

- Optional toppings: shredded carrots, sliced cucumbers, chopped cilantro, and a squeeze of lime juice

Instructions:

1. **Cook Turkey:** In a skillet, heat sesame oil over medium heat. Add onions, bell peppers, and garlic, and sauté until soft. Add ground turkey, soy sauce, and ginger. Cook until turkey is browned and cooked through.

2. **Assemble Wraps:** Spoon the cooked turkey mixture onto lettuce leaves. Add any optional toppings you like.

3. **Serve:** Fold the lettuce leaves over the filling and serve immediately.

Why It's Great: These wraps are low in carbs and high in protein, making them an ideal lunch option for those managing blood sugar levels. They're also light, refreshing, and full of flavor.

7. Cauliflower Rice with Stir-Fried Vegetables

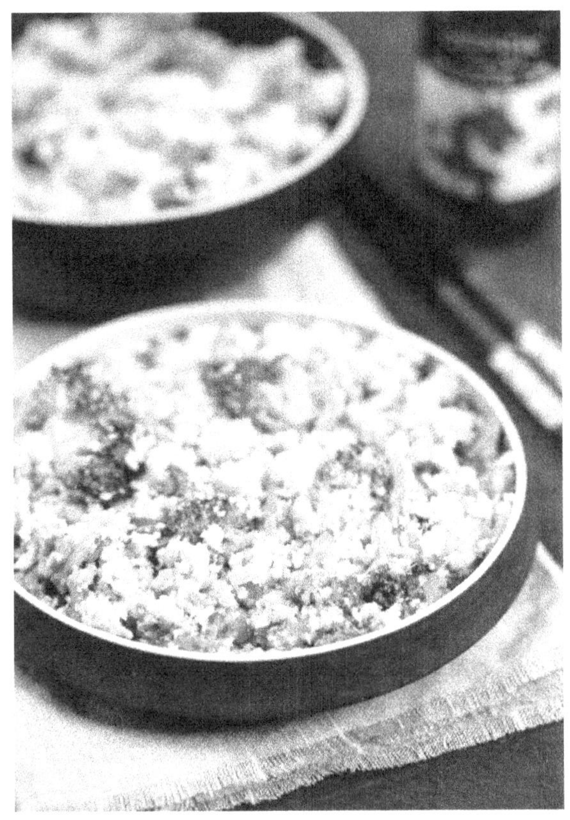

Description: Cauliflower Rice with Stir-Fried Vegetables is a low-carb alternative to traditional rice dishes. This meal is packed with colorful vegetables, offering a nutritious and satisfying lunch that's easy to prepare and perfect for those on a diabetes-friendly diet.

Ingredients:

- 1 small head of cauliflower, grated or processed into rice-sized pieces

- 1 cup broccoli florets

- 1/2 cup bell peppers, sliced

- 1/2 cup carrots, julienned

- 1/4 cup onions, chopped

- 2 tablespoons soy sauce or tamari

- 1 tablespoon olive oil

- 1 teaspoon sesame oil

- 1 clove garlic, minced

- 1 teaspoon ginger, grated

- Optional: sliced green onions and sesame seeds for garnish

Instructions:

1. **Prepare Cauliflower Rice:** Heat olive oil in a large skillet over medium heat. Add grated cauliflower and cook for 5-7 minutes until tender. Remove and set aside.

2. **Stir-Fry Vegetables:** In the same skillet, heat sesame oil. Add onions, garlic, and ginger, and sauté until fragrant. Add broccoli, bell peppers, and carrots, and stir-fry until vegetables are tender-crisp.

3. **Combine and Serve:** Return the cauliflower rice to the skillet with the vegetables. Add soy sauce and toss to combine. Garnish with green onions and sesame seeds if desired.

Why It's Great: Cauliflower rice is a great low-carb substitute for regular rice, and it pairs perfectly with stir-fried vegetables. This dish is full of fiber and vitamins, making it a nutritious and diabetes-friendly lunch option.

8. Caprese Salad with Balsamic Glaze

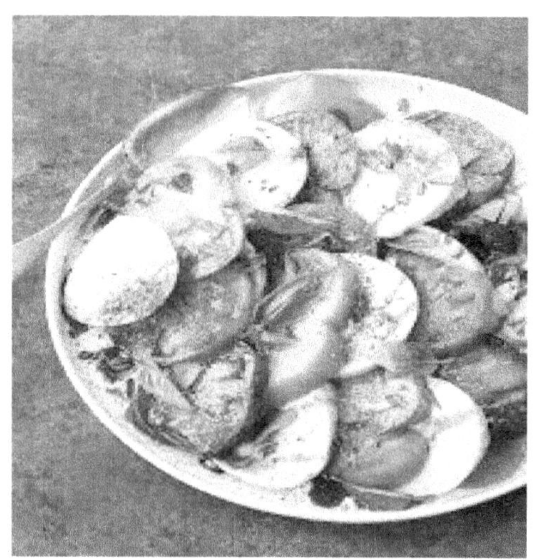

Description: Caprese Salad with Balsamic Glaze is a simple yet elegant dish that's perfect for a light lunch. The combination of fresh mozzarella, ripe tomatoes, and fragrant basil is refreshing, and the balsamic glaze adds a sweet and tangy finish.

Ingredients:

- 2 large ripe tomatoes, sliced

- 8 ounces fresh mozzarella, sliced

- 1/4 cup fresh basil leaves

- 2 tablespoons balsamic glaze

- 2 tablespoons olive oil

- Salt and pepper to taste

Instructions:

1. **Assemble Salad:** Arrange tomato and mozzarella slices on a platter, alternating them in a circle. Tuck fresh basil leaves between the slices.

2. **Dress Salad:** Drizzle with olive oil and balsamic glaze. Season with salt and pepper to taste.

3. **Serve:** Serve immediately as a light lunch or as a side dish.

Why It's Great: This salad is low in carbs and full of fresh flavors. The mozzarella provides a good source of protein, while the tomatoes and basil add antioxidants. The balsamic glaze ties everything together with a delightful sweetness.

9. Beef and Broccoli Stir-Fry

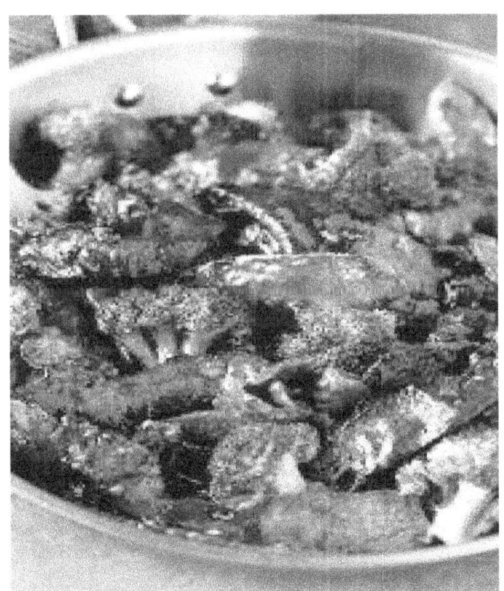

Description: Beef and Broccoli Stir-Fry is a classic dish that's both delicious and easy to prepare. This low-carb version skips the traditional sugary sauces and focuses on the natural flavors of the beef and broccoli, making it a great option for a diabetes-friendly lunch.

Ingredients:

- 1/2 pound flank steak, sliced thinly

- 2 cups broccoli florets

- 1/4 cup onions, sliced

- 2 tablespoons soy sauce or tamari

- 1 tablespoon sesame oil

- 1 teaspoon ginger, grated

- 2 cloves garlic, minced

- 1 tablespoon olive oil

- Optional: sesame seeds and sliced green onions for garnish

Instructions:

1. **Cook Beef:** In a large skillet or wok, heat olive oil over medium-high heat. Add sliced beef and cook until browned. Remove and set aside.

2. **Stir-Fry Vegetables:** In the same skillet, add sesame oil, onions, garlic, and ginger. Stir-fry until fragrant. Add broccoli and cook until tender-crisp.

3. **Combine and Serve:** Return the beef to the skillet and add soy sauce. Toss to combine and heat through. Garnish with sesame seeds and green onions if desired.

Why It's Great: This dish is rich in protein and low in carbs, making it ideal for maintaining stable blood sugar levels. The beef provides essential nutrients like iron, while the broccoli adds fiber and vitamins.

10. Low Carb Vegetable Soup with Chicken

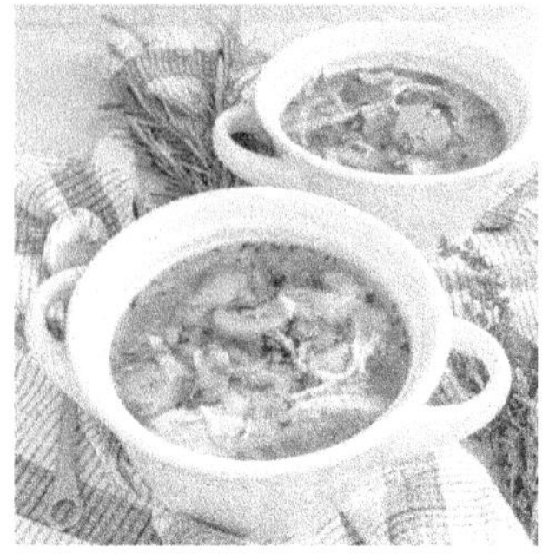

Description: Low Carb Vegetable Soup with Chicken is a comforting and nutritious lunch option that's perfect for any season. This soup is packed with a variety of vegetables and tender chicken, offering a filling meal that's low in carbs and full of flavor.

Ingredients:

- 1/2 pound chicken breast, cooked and shredded

- 4 cups chicken broth

- 1 cup zucchini, diced

- 1 cup celery, diced

- 1 cup carrots, diced

- 1/2 cup onions, chopped

- 2 cloves garlic, minced

- 1 teaspoon thyme

- 1 teaspoon oregano

- 1 tablespoon olive oil

- Salt and pepper to taste

- Optional: fresh parsley for garnish

Instructions:

1. **Sauté Vegetables:** In a large pot, heat olive oil over medium heat. Add onions, garlic, carrots, and celery. Sauté until vegetables are softened.

2. **Add Broth and Chicken:** Pour in chicken broth and add zucchini, thyme, and oregano. Bring to a boil, then reduce heat and simmer for 10-15 minutes.

3. **Add Chicken and Serve:** Stir in shredded chicken and cook until heated through. Season with salt and pepper. Garnish with fresh parsley if desired.

Why It's Great: This soup is low in carbs and high in fiber, making it a satisfying and diabetes-friendly lunch. The variety of vegetables provides a wide range of nutrients, while the chicken adds lean protein to keep you full and energized.

These lunch recipes offer a range of flavors and textures, ensuring that you have plenty of delicious options to choose from. Each dish is designed to be low in carbs and sugar, making them ideal for maintaining stable blood sugar levels while still enjoying a satisfying meal. Whether you prefer a light salad, a hearty wrap, or a comforting soup, these recipes have you covered.

CHAPTER 4

DINNER RECIPES

Dinner is more than just a meal—it's a time to unwind, nourish your body, and connect with loved ones after a long day. For individuals managing diabetes, dinner can also be a crucial part of maintaining stable blood sugar levels and overall health. This collection of dinner recipes is designed to make that task easier and more enjoyable, offering a variety of flavorful, satisfying, and diabetes-friendly dishes that are low in carbs and sugar.

These recipes are crafted with both taste and nutrition in mind, ensuring that you don't have to sacrifice flavor for health. Whether you're in the mood for a quick weeknight meal or a more elaborate dish to share with family and friends, you'll find something here to suit your needs. From hearty proteins like baked salmon and grilled pork chops to vibrant vegetables and creative low-carb substitutes like zoodles and cauliflower mash, these dinners are both delicious and nourishing.

Each recipe is carefully designed to help you manage your diabetes while still enjoying a rich and varied diet. The ingredients are chosen to provide essential nutrients, promote satiety, and minimize blood sugar spikes, making these meals a valuable part of a balanced diet. Whether you're cooking for yourself or for a crowd, these recipes offer something for everyone, ensuring that dinner remains a pleasurable and healthful experience.

So, get ready to explore a world of culinary possibilities that not only support your health but also satisfy your taste buds. These dinner recipes are more than just meals—they're a pathway to better living, one delicious bite at a time.

1. Baked Salmon with Asparagus

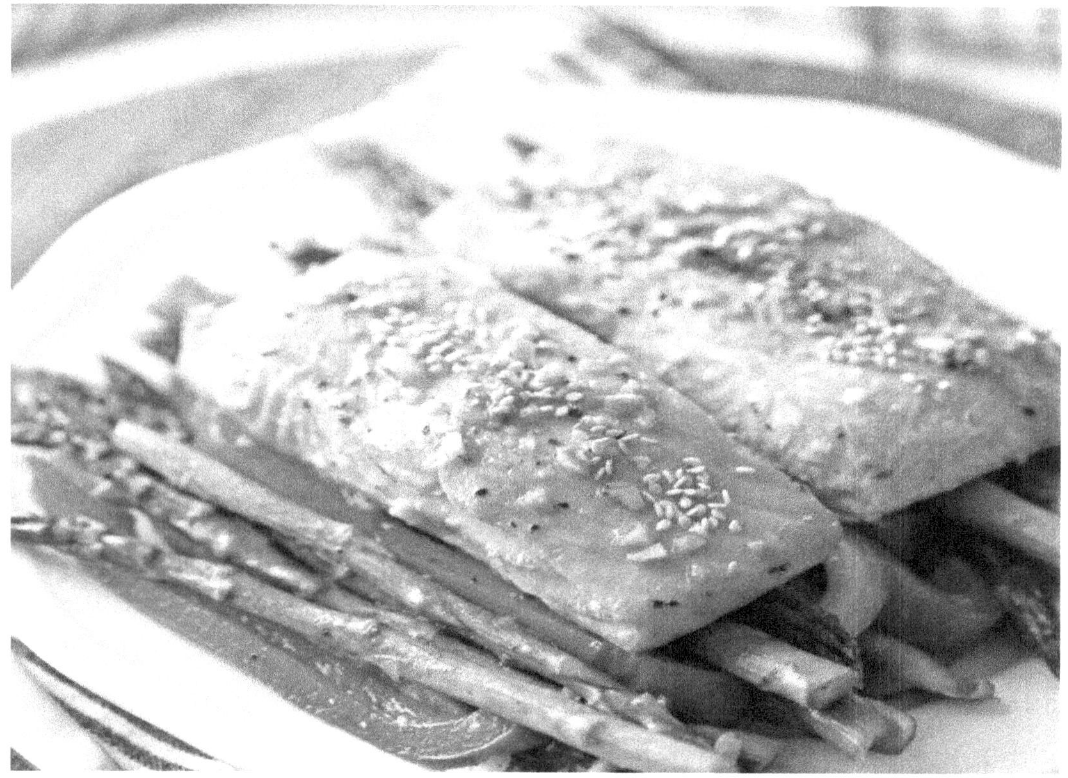

Description: Baked Salmon with Asparagus is a simple and nutritious dinner that's perfect for any night of the week. This dish is packed with omega-3 fatty acids from the salmon and fiber from the asparagus, making it both heart-healthy and diabetes-friendly.

Ingredients:

- 2 salmon fillets

- 1 bunch asparagus, trimmed

- 2 tablespoons olive oil

- 1 lemon, sliced

- 2 cloves garlic, minced

- Salt and pepper to taste

- Optional: fresh dill or parsley for garnish

Instructions:

1. **Prepare the Baking Sheet:** Preheat your oven to 400°F (200°C). Line a baking sheet with parchment paper.

2. **Season the Salmon:** Place salmon fillets on the baking sheet. Drizzle with olive oil, and season with minced garlic, salt, and pepper. Arrange lemon slices on top of the salmon.

3. **Add Asparagus:** Place the asparagus around the salmon on the baking sheet. Drizzle with olive oil and season with salt and pepper.

4. **Bake:** Bake in the preheated oven for 12-15 minutes, or until the salmon is cooked through and the asparagus is tender.

5. **Serve:** Garnish with fresh dill or parsley if desired, and serve immediately.

Why It's Great: This dish is quick to prepare and full of flavor. Salmon is a great source of healthy fats and protein, while asparagus adds fiber and essential vitamins. It's a well-balanced, low-carb dinner option.

2. Stuffed Bell Peppers with Ground Turkey

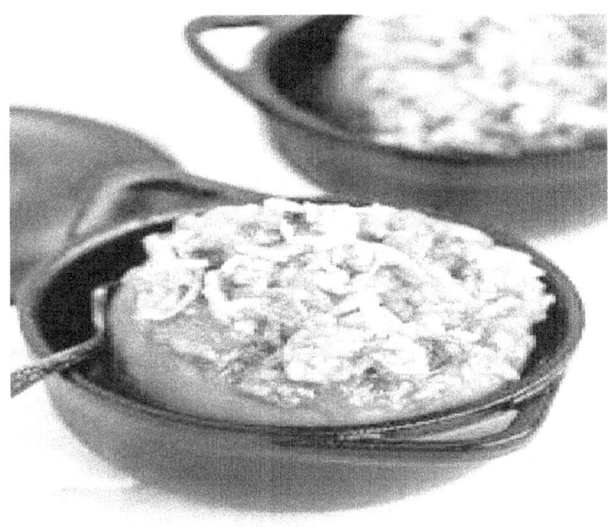

Description: Stuffed Bell Peppers with Ground Turkey are a satisfying and colorful dinner option. The peppers are filled with a savory mixture of ground turkey, vegetables, and spices, making it a delicious and healthy meal.

Ingredients:

- 4 bell peppers, tops cut off and seeds removed

- 1 pound ground turkey

- 1 cup cauliflower rice

- 1/2 cup onions, chopped

- 1/2 cup tomatoes, diced

- 1/2 cup shredded cheese (optional)

- 2 cloves garlic, minced

- 1 teaspoon Italian seasoning

- 2 tablespoons olive oil

- Salt and pepper to taste

Instructions:

1. **Preheat Oven:** Preheat your oven to 375°F (190°C).

2. **Cook the Filling:** In a large skillet, heat olive oil over medium heat. Add onions and garlic, and sauté until softened. Add ground turkey, Italian seasoning, salt, and pepper, and cook until the turkey is browned. Stir in cauliflower rice and tomatoes, and cook for another 2-3 minutes.

3. **Stuff the Peppers:** Stuff each bell pepper with the turkey mixture. Place the stuffed peppers in a baking dish and cover with foil.

4. **Bake:** Bake in the preheated oven for 25-30 minutes. If using cheese, uncover the dish and sprinkle cheese on top in the last 5 minutes of baking.

5. **Serve:** Serve hot, garnished with fresh herbs if desired.

Why It's Great: This dish is packed with protein and vegetables, making it a filling and nutritious option for dinner. The ground turkey is lean and flavorful, while the bell peppers add a sweet and crunchy texture.

3. Garlic Butter Steak Bites with Green Beans

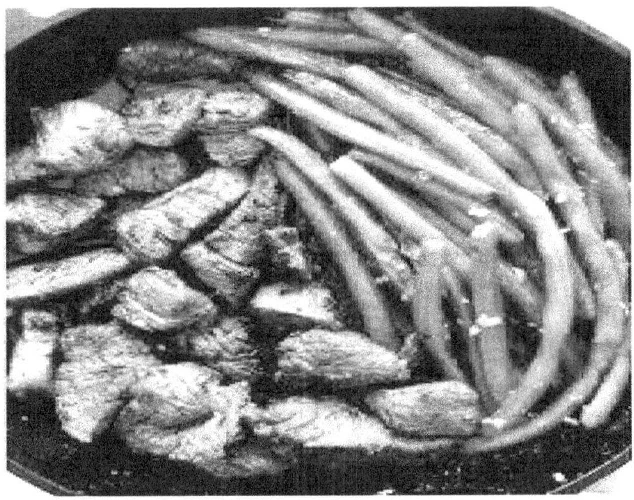

Description: Garlic Butter Steak Bites with Green Beans is a hearty and flavorful dinner that's sure to satisfy. The steak bites are tender and juicy, while the green beans add a fresh and crisp contrast.

Ingredients:

- 1 pound steak (sirloin or ribeye), cut into bite-sized pieces

- 2 cups green beans, trimmed

- 3 tablespoons butter

- 3 cloves garlic, minced

- 1 tablespoon olive oil

- Salt and pepper to taste

- Optional: fresh parsley for garnish

Instructions:

1. **Cook the Steak Bites:** In a large skillet, heat olive oil over medium-high heat. Add steak bites and season with salt and pepper. Cook for 2-3 minutes per side until browned and cooked to your liking. Remove from the skillet and set aside.

2. **Cook the Green Beans:** In the same skillet, add butter and minced garlic. Sauté for 1-2 minutes until fragrant. Add green beans and cook until tender, about 5-7 minutes.

3. **Combine and Serve:** Return the steak bites to the skillet and toss with the green beans. Cook for an additional 1-2 minutes to heat through. Garnish with fresh parsley if desired, and serve immediately.

Why It's Great: This dish is rich in protein and low in carbs, making it an excellent option for a diabetes-friendly dinner. The garlic butter adds a delicious flavor to both the steak and the green beans.

4. Low Carb Chicken Parmesan

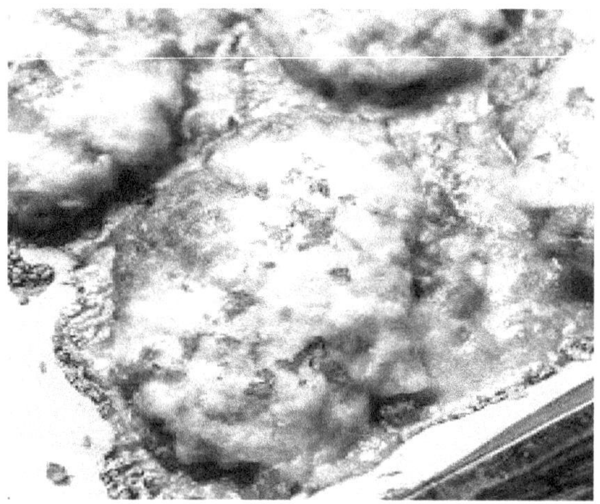

Description: Low Carb Chicken Parmesan is a lighter take on the classic Italian dish. Instead of breading the chicken, this version uses a flavorful coating of Parmesan cheese, making it both low-carb and packed with flavor.

Ingredients:

- 2 chicken breasts, pounded thin

- 1/2 cup grated Parmesan cheese

- 1/2 cup marinara sauce

- 1/2 cup shredded mozzarella cheese

- 1 teaspoon Italian seasoning

- 2 tablespoons olive oil

- Salt and pepper to taste

- Optional: fresh basil for garnish

Instructions:

1. **Preheat Oven:** Preheat your oven to 400°F (200°C).

2. **Prepare the Chicken:** Season the chicken breasts with salt, pepper, and Italian seasoning. Coat each chicken breast with grated Parmesan cheese.

3. **Cook the Chicken:** In a large oven-safe skillet, heat olive oil over medium-high heat. Add the chicken and cook for 2-3 minutes per side until golden brown.

4. **Bake:** Top each chicken breast with marinara sauce and shredded mozzarella cheese. Transfer the skillet to the oven and bake for 10-15 minutes until the cheese is melted and bubbly.

5. **Serve:** Garnish with fresh basil if desired, and serve hot.

Why It's Great: This dish is a satisfying and low-carb alternative to traditional Chicken Parmesan. The Parmesan coating adds a rich flavor, while the marinara sauce provides a tangy contrast.

5. Lemon Herb Roasted Chicken with Brussels Sprouts

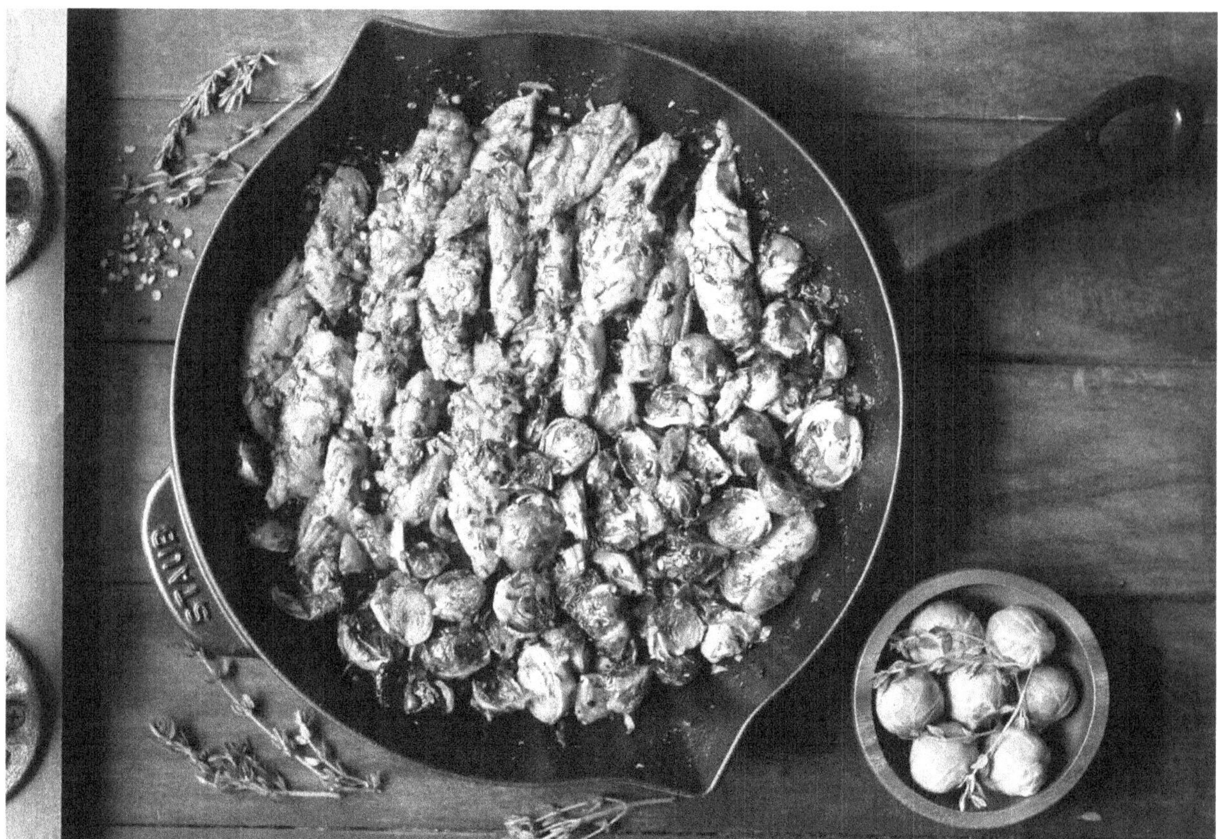

Description: Lemon Herb Roasted Chicken with Brussels Sprouts is a flavorful and easy-to-make dinner that's perfect for a weeknight meal. The chicken is marinated in a lemon-herb mixture, while the Brussels sprouts are roasted to perfection.

Ingredients:

- 4 chicken thighs, bone-in and skin-on

- 1 pound Brussels sprouts, trimmed and halved

- 2 lemons, juiced and zested

- 3 cloves garlic, minced

- 2 tablespoons olive oil

- 1 teaspoon thyme

- 1 teaspoon rosemary

- Salt and pepper to taste

Instructions:

1. **Marinate the Chicken:** In a large bowl, combine lemon juice, zest, garlic, thyme, rosemary, olive oil, salt, and pepper. Add chicken thighs and marinate for at least 30 minutes.

2. **Preheat Oven:** Preheat your oven to 400°F (200°C).

3. **Roast the Chicken and Brussels Sprouts:** Place marinated chicken thighs on a baking sheet. Toss Brussels sprouts in the remaining marinade and arrange them around the chicken. Roast for 30-35 minutes until the chicken is cooked through and the Brussels sprouts are tender and caramelized.

4. **Serve:** Serve hot, garnished with lemon slices if desired.

Why It's Great: This dish is packed with flavor and nutrients. The chicken is juicy and aromatic, while the Brussels sprouts add a delicious crunch. It's a perfect low-carb, high-protein dinner.

6. Grilled Pork Chops with Cauliflower Mash

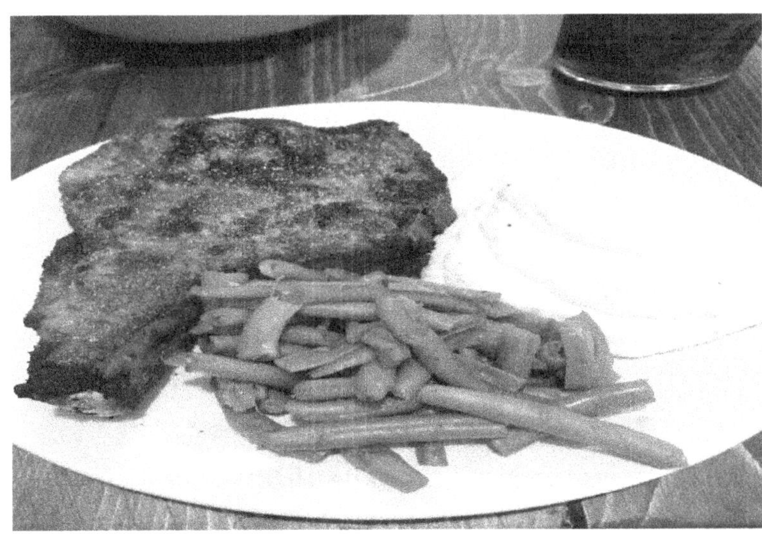

Description: Grilled Pork Chops with Cauliflower Mash is a satisfying and comforting dinner. The pork chops are perfectly seasoned and grilled, while the cauliflower mash is a low-carb alternative to traditional mashed potatoes.

Ingredients:

- 4 pork chops

- 1 head cauliflower, cut into florets

- 1/4 cup heavy cream

- 2 tablespoons butter

- 2 cloves garlic, minced

- 1 teaspoon paprika

- 1 teaspoon garlic powder

- Salt and pepper to taste

- Optional: fresh chives for garnish

Instructions:

1. **Season the Pork Chops:** Season pork chops with paprika, garlic powder, salt, and pepper.

2. **Grill the Pork Chops:** Preheat your grill to medium-high heat. Grill pork chops for 4-5 minutes per side until cooked through.

3. **Make the Cauliflower Mash:** In a large pot, bring cauliflower florets to a boil in salted water. Cook until tender, about 10 minutes. Drain and mash with butter, heavy cream, and minced garlic. Season with salt and pepper.

4. **Serve:** Serve the grilled pork chops with a side of cauliflower mash. Garnish with fresh chives if desired.

Why It's Great: This dish is rich in protein and low in carbs, making it ideal for a diabetes-friendly dinner. The cauliflower mash is creamy and delicious, providing a great alternative to potatoes.

7. Zoodles with Meatballs in Marinara Sauce

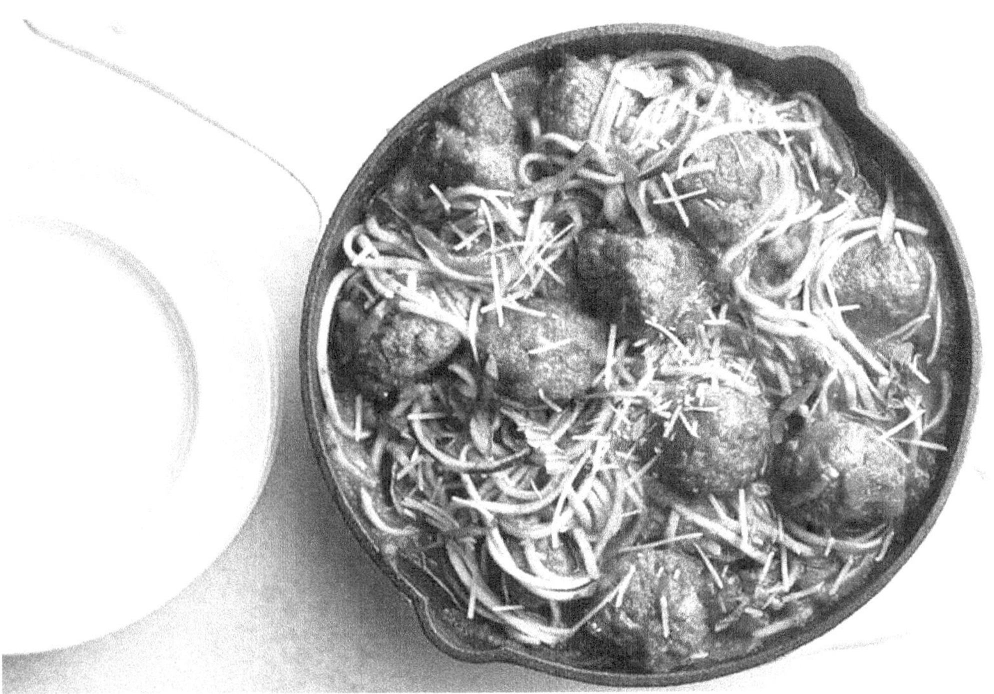

Description: Zoodles with Meatballs in Marinara Sauce is a low-carb twist on a classic Italian dish. Zucchini noodles (zoodles) are a great substitute for pasta, and they pair perfectly with tender meatballs and marinara sauce.

Ingredients:

- 4 zucchini, spiralized into noodles

- 1 pound ground beef or turkey

- 1/4 cup Parmesan cheese, grated

- 1/4 cup almond flour

- 1 egg

- 1/2 teaspoon garlic powder

- 1/2 teaspoon onion powder

- 1 teaspoon Italian seasoning

- 2 cups marinara sauce

- 2 tablespoons olive oil

- Salt and pepper to taste

- Optional: fresh basil for garnish

Instructions:

1. **Make the Meatballs:** In a large bowl, combine ground meat, Parmesan cheese, almond flour, egg, garlic powder, onion powder, Italian seasoning, salt, and pepper. Form into meatballs.

2. **Cook the Meatballs:** In a large skillet, heat olive oil over medium heat. Add meatballs and cook until browned on all sides. Remove from the skillet and set aside.

3. **Prepare the Zoodles:** In the same skillet, add zoodles and sauté for 2-3 minutes until slightly softened. Remove and set aside.

4. **Simmer the Sauce:** Add marinara sauce to the skillet and bring to a simmer. Return meatballs to the skillet and cook until heated through.

5. **Serve:** Serve the meatballs over zoodles, garnished with fresh basil if desired.

Why It's Great: This dish is a delicious and low-carb alternative to traditional spaghetti and meatballs. The zoodles are light and refreshing, while the meatballs are full of flavor.

8. Shrimp Scampi with Zucchini Noodles

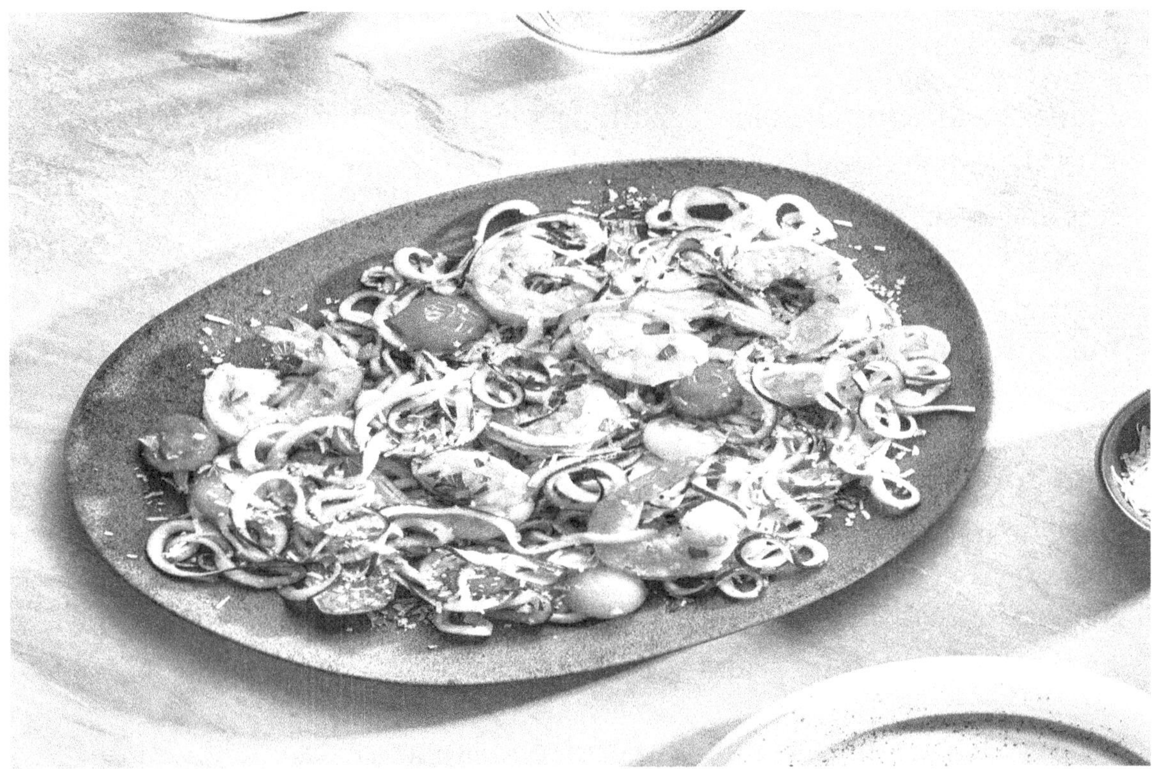

Description: Shrimp Scampi with Zucchini Noodles is a light and flavorful dinner that's perfect for a low-carb diet. The shrimp are cooked in a garlic butter sauce and served over zoodles for a fresh and satisfying meal.

Ingredients:

- 1 pound shrimp, peeled and deveined

- 4 zucchini, spiralized into noodles

- 3 cloves garlic, minced

- 1/4 cup butter

- 1/4 cup white wine or chicken broth

- 1 tablespoon lemon juice

- 1 tablespoon olive oil

- Salt and pepper to taste

- Optional: fresh parsley for garnish

Instructions:

1. **Cook the Shrimp:** In a large skillet, heat olive oil over medium heat. Add shrimp and cook until pink and opaque, about 2-3 minutes per side. Remove from the skillet and set aside.

2. **Make the Scampi Sauce:** In the same skillet, melt butter and add minced garlic. Sauté until fragrant. Add white wine or chicken broth and lemon juice, and simmer for 2-3 minutes.

3. **Add Zoodles:** Add zoodles to the skillet and toss in the scampi sauce until heated through, about 2 minutes.

4. **Serve:** Return shrimp to the skillet and toss to combine. Garnish with fresh parsley if desired, and serve immediately.

Why It's Great: This dish is light, flavorful, and low in carbs, making it an ideal dinner for those managing diabetes. The garlic butter sauce pairs perfectly with the shrimp and zoodles, creating a satisfying meal.

9. Herb-Crusted Cod with Steamed Broccoli

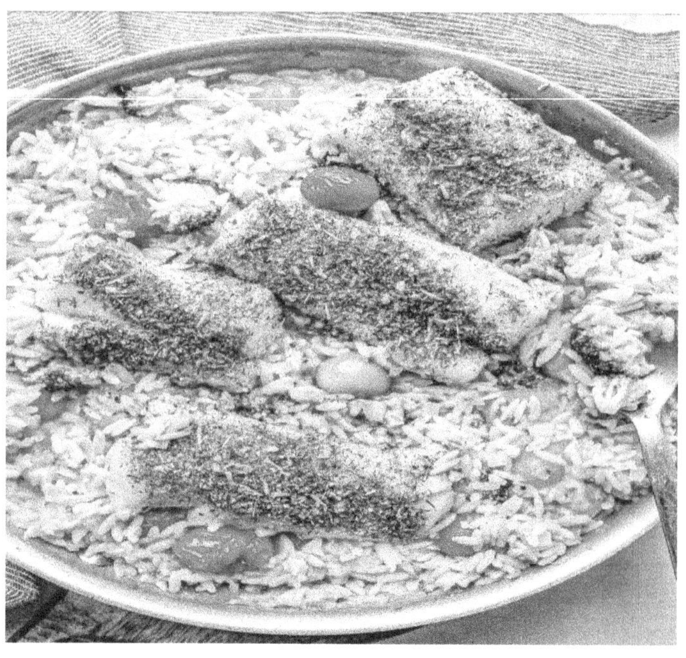

Description: Herb-Crusted Cod with Steamed Broccoli is a healthy and delicious dinner that's easy to make. The cod is coated in a flavorful herb crust, while the broccoli is steamed to perfection, making this dish both nutritious and satisfying.

Ingredients:

- 2 cod fillets
- 1/2 cup almond flour
- 1/4 cup Parmesan cheese, grated
- 1 tablespoon fresh parsley, chopped
- 1 teaspoon thyme
- 1 teaspoon garlic powder
- 1/2 teaspoon paprika
- 2 tablespoons olive oil
- 2 cups broccoli florets
- Salt and pepper to taste
- Optional: lemon wedges for serving

Instructions:

1. **Preheat Oven:** Preheat your oven to 400°F (200°C).

2. **Prepare the Herb Crust:** In a small bowl, combine almond flour, Parmesan cheese, parsley, thyme, garlic powder, paprika, salt, and pepper. Coat each cod fillet with the mixture.

3. **Bake the Cod:** Place the coated cod fillets on a baking sheet lined with parchment paper. Drizzle with olive oil and bake for 12-15 minutes until the fish is cooked through and the crust is golden.

4. **Steam the Broccoli:** While the fish is baking, steam the broccoli until tender.

5. **Serve:** Serve the herb-crusted cod with steamed broccoli and lemon wedges on the side.

Why It's Great: This dish is rich in protein and low in carbs, making it a great choice for a diabetes-friendly dinner. The herb crust adds a delicious flavor to the cod, while the steamed broccoli provides a healthy and fiber-rich side.

10. Eggplant Lasagna

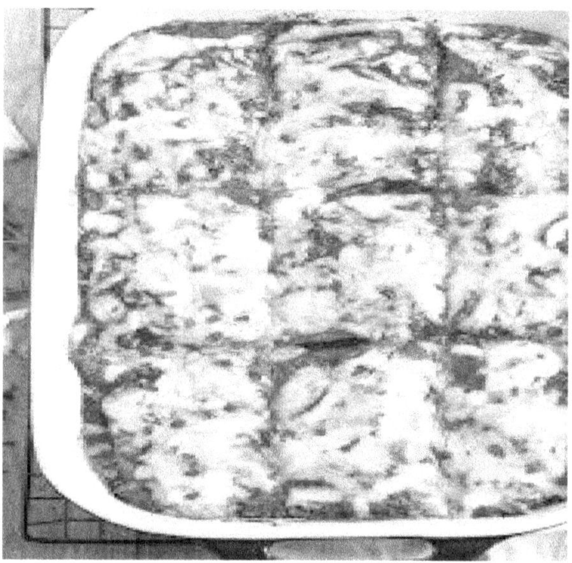

Description: Eggplant Lasagna is a low-carb and vegetarian alternative to traditional lasagna. Layers of roasted eggplant replace pasta, while a rich tomato sauce and cheesy filling make this dish just as satisfying as the original.

Ingredients:

- 2 large eggplants, sliced lengthwise

- 2 cups marinara sauce

- 1 cup ricotta cheese

- 1 cup mozzarella cheese, shredded

- 1/4 cup Parmesan cheese, grated

- 1 egg

- 1 teaspoon Italian seasoning

- 2 tablespoons olive oil

- Salt and pepper to taste

- Optional: fresh basil for garnish

Instructions:

1. **Preheat Oven:** Preheat your oven to 375°F (190°C).

2. **Prepare the Eggplant:** Brush eggplant slices with olive oil and season with salt and pepper. Roast on a baking sheet for 15-20 minutes until tender.

3. **Mix the Filling:** In a bowl, combine ricotta cheese, Parmesan cheese, egg, Italian seasoning, salt, and pepper.

4. **Assemble the Lasagna:** In a baking dish, spread a layer of marinara sauce. Add a layer of roasted eggplant slices, followed by a layer of the ricotta mixture. Repeat the layers, ending with a layer of marinara sauce and shredded mozzarella cheese.

5. **Bake:** Bake in the preheated oven for 25-30 minutes until the cheese is melted and bubbly.

6. **Serve:** Garnish with fresh basil if desired, and serve hot.

Why It's Great: This Eggplant Lasagna is a delicious and low-carb alternative to traditional lasagna. The eggplant provides a hearty texture, while the cheesy filling makes this dish comforting and satisfying.

These dinner recipes offer a variety of flavors and textures, ensuring that you have plenty of delicious options to choose from. Each dish is designed to be low in carbs and sugar, making them ideal for maintaining stable blood sugar levels while still enjoying a satisfying meal. Whether you prefer seafood, poultry, or vegetarian dishes, these recipes have you covered.

CHAPTER 5

SNACK IDEAS

When managing diabetes, it's essential to choose snacks that are low in sugar and carbohydrates while still providing satisfaction and energy. The following snack ideas are designed to meet these criteria, offering a variety of flavors and textures to keep your taste buds excited and your blood sugar stable.

1. Almonds and Cheese

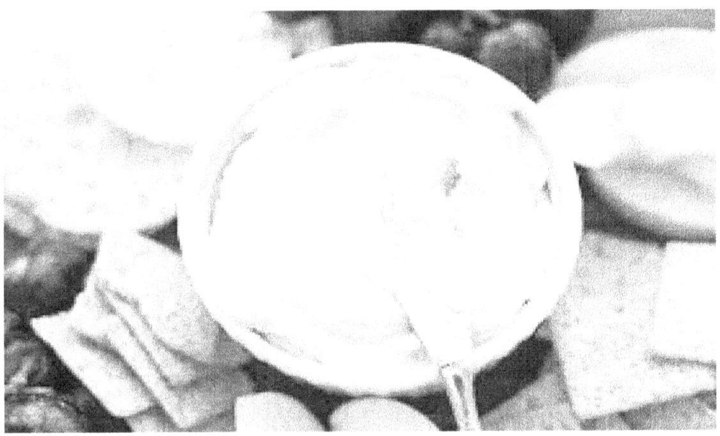

Description: Almonds and cheese form a delightful combination that merges the crunch of almonds with the creamy richness of cheese. This snack is not only tasty but also highly nutritious. Almonds are packed with monounsaturated fats, fiber, and protein, which contribute to heart health and stable blood sugar levels. Cheese adds a creamy, satisfying element and additional protein, which further helps in managing hunger and blood sugar.

Ingredients:

- **1 small handful of raw almonds (about 1 ounce):** Rich in healthy fats, fiber, and protein, almonds are a great choice for a satisfying snack.

- **2-3 slices or cubes of cheese (cheddar, gouda, or mozzarella):** Cheese provides a creamy texture and additional protein, complementing the almonds perfectly.

Instructions:

1. **Prepare the Almonds:** Measure out a small handful of raw almonds. You can opt for plain almonds or those lightly salted, depending on your preference.

2. **Slice the Cheese:** Choose your favorite type of cheese and slice or cube it into bite-sized pieces.

3. **Combine and Serve:** Arrange the almonds and cheese on a plate or in a snack container. This snack can be enjoyed immediately or packed for later.

Why It's Great: Almonds and cheese offer a satisfying crunch and creamy texture, making them a delicious and filling option. The combination of protein and healthy fats helps to keep you full and maintain stable blood sugar levels. This snack is also easy to prepare and perfect for on-the-go eating.

Nutritional Benefits:

- **Almonds:** Provide healthy fats, fiber, vitamin E, and magnesium. They help regulate blood sugar and support cardiovascular health.

- **Cheese:** Adds protein and calcium, essential for bone health and muscle function.

Variations:

- **Flavored Almonds:** Try using flavored almonds, such as those with rosemary or garlic, for a different taste experience.

- **Cheese Types:** Experiment with various types of cheese like goat cheese, provolone, or Swiss for a change in flavor.

2. Cucumber Slices with Hummus

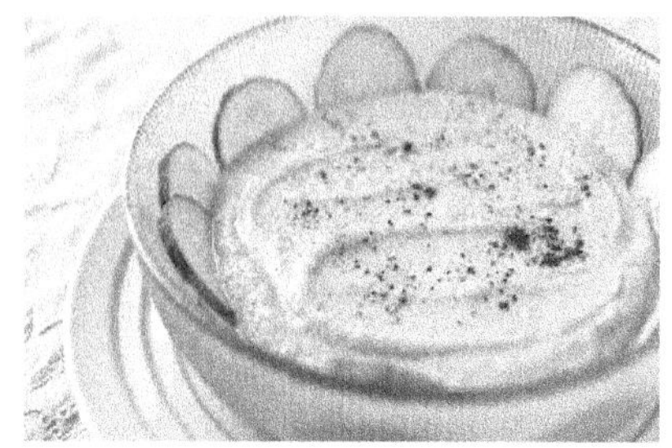

Description: Cucumber slices with hummus offer a refreshing and hydrating snack. Cucumbers are low in calories and carbohydrates while providing a crisp texture. Hummus, made from chickpeas and tahini, adds a creamy, protein-rich element that makes this snack both satisfying and nutritious.

Ingredients:

- **1 cucumber:** Sliced into rounds or sticks, cucumbers are hydrating and low in carbs.

- **1/2 cup hummus:** Choose store-bought or homemade hummus. Look for versions with minimal added sugars and healthy oils.

Instructions:

1. **Prepare the Cucumber:** Wash the cucumber thoroughly. Slice it into thin rounds or sticks based on your preference.

2. **Serve with Hummus:** Place the cucumber slices on a plate and serve with a side of hummus for dipping.

Why It's Great: This snack is light yet filling, with cucumbers offering a refreshing crunch and hummus providing a rich, creamy dip. It's perfect for a quick snack that supports hydration and provides a good mix of protein and fiber.

Nutritional Benefits:

- **Cucumbers:** Low in calories and carbohydrates, high in water content. They aid in hydration and offer a mild, refreshing flavor.

- **Hummus:** Contains protein, fiber, and healthy fats from chickpeas and tahini, supporting satiety and digestive health.

Variations:

- **Flavored Hummus:** Experiment with different hummus flavors such as roasted red pepper, spicy harissa, or garlic.

- **Herbed Cucumbers:** Sprinkle cucumber slices with fresh herbs like dill or mint for added flavor.

3. Celery Sticks with Peanut Butter

Description: Celery sticks with peanut butter create a crunchy and creamy snack that's both satisfying and nutritious. Celery provides a crisp texture and minimal carbs, while peanut butter adds protein and healthy fats. This classic combination is not only delicious but also supports stable blood sugar levels.

Ingredients:

- **2-3 celery stalks:** Cut into sticks, celery is low in calories and provides a satisfying crunch.

- **2 tablespoons natural peanut butter:** Choose peanut butter without added sugars or hydrogenated oils.

Instructions:

1. **Prepare the Celery:** Wash and cut the celery stalks into sticks, ensuring they are of a suitable size for dipping.

2. **Spread the Peanut Butter:** Spoon peanut butter onto each celery stick or serve it on the side for dipping.

Why It's Great: This snack offers a satisfying crunch from the celery and a creamy, rich taste from the peanut butter. It's a great source of protein and healthy fats, helping to keep you full and maintain stable blood sugar levels.

Nutritional Benefits:

- **Celery:** Provides fiber and hydration with minimal calories and carbohydrates.

- **Peanut Butter:** Offers protein, healthy fats, and a small amount of fiber, supporting satiety and energy levels.

Variations:

- **Almond Butter:** Substitute almond butter for a different nutty flavor and additional nutrients.

- **Celery with Other Toppings:** Top celery with other spreads like sunflower seed butter or Greek yogurt for variety.

4. Hard-Boiled Eggs with a Dash of Hot Sauce

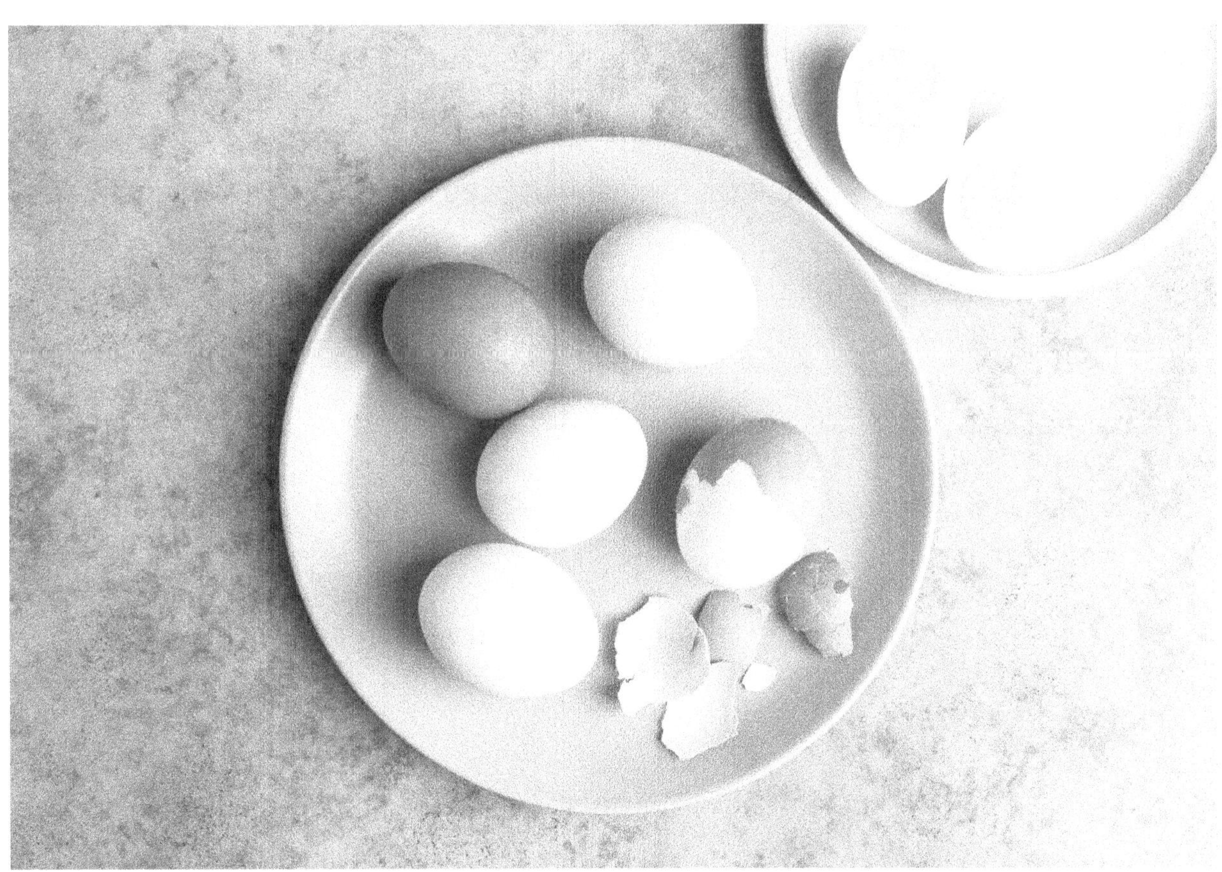

Description: Hard-boiled eggs with a dash of hot sauce are a protein-packed snack with a spicy kick. Eggs are an excellent source of high-quality protein, vitamins, and minerals. The addition of hot sauce adds flavor without additional carbs or calories.

Ingredients:

- **2 hard-boiled eggs:** Cooked and peeled, eggs are an easy source of protein.

- **A few dashes of hot sauce:** Choose your favorite hot sauce to add a bit of spice.

Instructions:

1. **Prepare the Eggs:** Boil eggs until they are hard (about 10 minutes). Cool them, peel, and slice in half.

2. **Season with Hot Sauce:** Sprinkle or dash hot sauce over the eggs according to your taste.

Why It's Great: Hard-boiled eggs are easy to prepare and store, making them a convenient and portable snack. The hot sauce adds a flavorful kick without adding extra carbs, making this a great option for those who enjoy a bit of spice.

Nutritional Benefits:

- **Eggs:** Rich in protein, vitamins A, D, and B12, and minerals like selenium and choline.

- **Hot Sauce:** Adds flavor without significant calories or carbs.

Variations:

- **Spiced Eggs:** Experiment with other seasonings like paprika, cayenne pepper, or garlic powder.

- **Stuffed Eggs:** Try stuffing the egg whites with a mixture of avocado and spices for added flavor.

5. Greek Yogurt with Nuts and Seeds

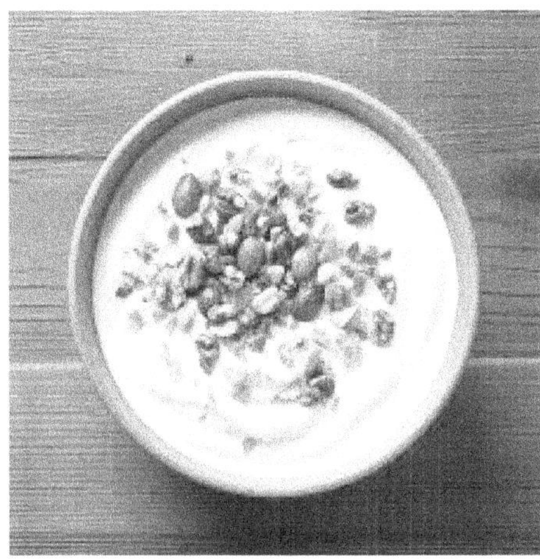

Description: Greek yogurt with nuts and seeds combines the creamy texture of Greek yogurt with the crunch of nuts and seeds. Greek yogurt is high in protein and probiotics, which support digestive health, while nuts and seeds add a satisfying crunch and additional nutrients.

Ingredients:

- **1 cup plain Greek yogurt:** High in protein and probiotics, providing a creamy base.

- **2 tablespoons mixed nuts:** Choose from almonds, walnuts, or pecans for variety.

- **1 tablespoon chia seeds or flaxseeds:** Add for extra fiber and omega-3 fatty acids.

Instructions:

1. **Prepare the Yogurt:** Spoon Greek yogurt into a bowl.

2. **Top with Nuts and Seeds:** Sprinkle mixed nuts and chia or flaxseeds on top of the yogurt.

Why It's Great: This snack provides a rich source of protein and healthy fats, keeping you full and supporting stable blood sugar levels. The combination of creamy yogurt with crunchy nuts and seeds offers a satisfying texture and flavor.

Nutritional Benefits:

- **Greek Yogurt:** Offers protein, calcium, and probiotics for digestive health.

- **Nuts and Seeds:** Provide healthy fats, fiber, and essential nutrients like omega-3 fatty acids.

Variations:

- **Fruit Additions:** Add fresh berries or a small amount of low-carb fruit for added flavor.

- **Spices:** Experiment with cinnamon or a touch of vanilla extract for extra flavor.

6. Guacamole with Veggie Sticks

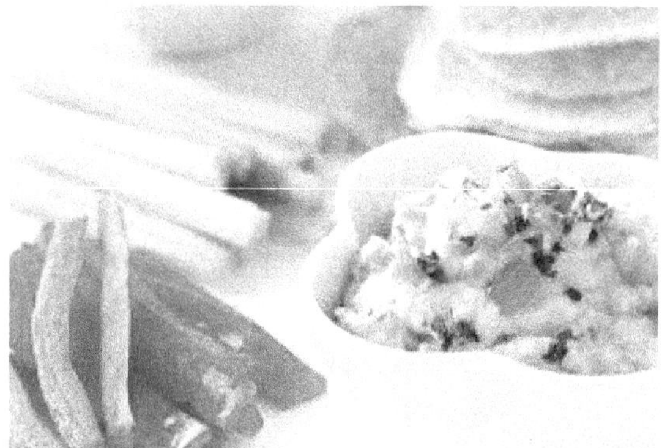

Description: Guacamole with veggie sticks is a nutrient-dense snack that pairs the creamy, flavorful guacamole with crisp, crunchy vegetables. Guacamole, made from avocados, provides healthy fats and a smooth texture, while veggie sticks add a refreshing crunch.

Ingredients:

- **1 cup guacamole:** Homemade or store-bought, with minimal added sugars and preservatives.

- **Assorted veggie sticks:** Use bell peppers, carrots, cucumbers, or celery sticks.

Instructions:

1. **Prepare the Vegetables:** Slice vegetables into sticks or bite-sized pieces.

2. **Serve with Guacamole:** Place the veggie sticks on a plate and serve with guacamole for dipping.

Why It's Great: Guacamole provides a creamy, flavorful dip that complements the crunch of fresh vegetables. This snack is packed with nutrients and healthy fats, making it both satisfying and beneficial for blood sugar control.

Nutritional Benefits:

- **Guacamole:** Rich in healthy fats, vitamins E and C, and potassium from avocados.

- **Veggie Sticks:** Low in calories and carbs, providing fiber and essential vitamins.

Variations:

- **Guacamole Add-ins:** Add chopped tomatoes, onions, or cilantro to your guacamole for added flavor.

- **Veggie Choices:** Try different vegetables like radishes or snap peas for variety.

7. Low Carb Cheese Crackers

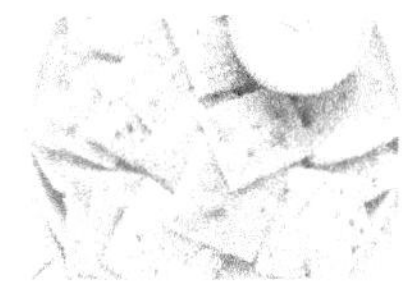

Description: Low-carb cheese crackers offer a crunchy, savory snack that's a great alternative to traditional high-carb crackers. Made with cheese and almond flour, these crackers are perfect for satisfying your craving for something crispy and cheesy without the carbs.

Ingredients:

- **1 cup shredded cheddar cheese:** Provides the base for the crackers.

- **1/2 cup almond flour:** A low-carb alternative to regular flour.

- **1/2 teaspoon paprika or your favorite seasoning:** For added flavor.

Instructions:

1. **Preheat Oven:** Set your oven to 350°F (175°C).

2. **Mix Ingredients:** In a bowl, combine shredded cheese, almond flour, and seasoning.

3. **Shape the Crackers:** Drop spoonfuls of the mixture onto a baking sheet and flatten with the back of a spoon.

4. **Bake:** Cook for 10-12 minutes, or until golden brown and crispy.

5. **Cool and Serve:** Allow to cool before serving.

Why It's Great: These cheese crackers are a low-carb, protein-rich option that provides a satisfying crunch. They are easy to make and perfect for snacking between meals.

Nutritional Benefits:

- **Cheese:** Offers protein and calcium, contributing to bone health and satiety.

- **Almond Flour:** Low in carbs and provides fiber and healthy fats.

Variations:

- **Cheese Varieties:** Experiment with different cheeses like Parmesan or Gouda for varied flavors.

- **Seasonings:** Try different herbs and spices like garlic powder or dried rosemary.

8. Tuna Salad Lettuce Boats

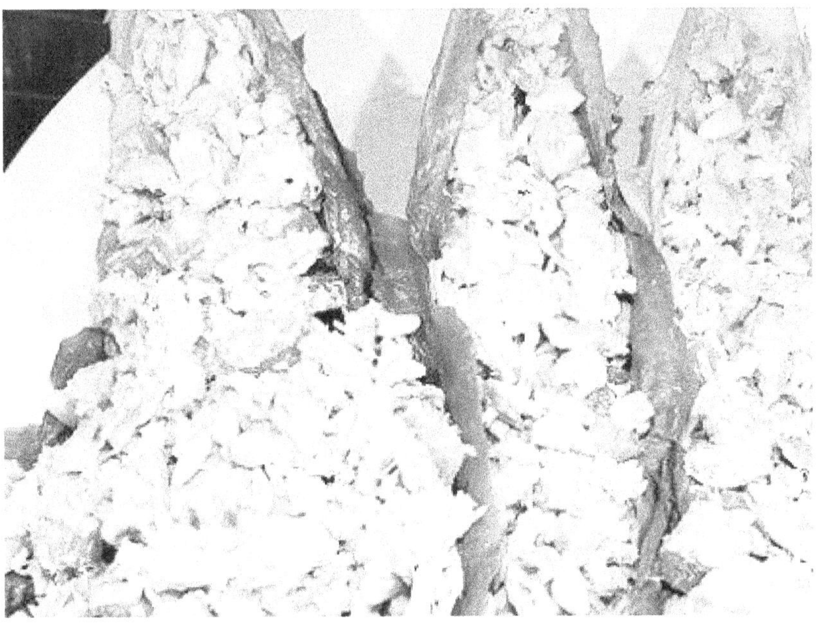

Description: Tuna salad lettuce boats are a convenient and protein-rich snack that replaces traditional bread with crisp lettuce leaves. The tuna salad, made with a simple mix of tuna, mayonnaise, and seasonings, is served in lettuce leaves, making it a low-carb, satisfying option.

Ingredients:

- **1 can of tuna:** Drained and flaked.

- **2 tablespoons mayonnaise:** Use a low-carb variety if preferred.

- **1 tablespoon chopped celery:** For added crunch and flavor.

- **1 teaspoon mustard:** Adds a tangy flavor.

- **Salt and pepper to taste**

- **4 large lettuce leaves:** Romaine or Butter lettuce works well.

Instructions:

1. **Prepare the Tuna Salad:** In a bowl, mix together the drained tuna, mayonnaise, chopped celery, mustard, salt, and pepper.

2. **Assemble the Boats:** Spoon the tuna salad onto the lettuce leaves, creating boats.

3. **Serve:** Enjoy immediately or refrigerate until ready to eat.

Why It's Great: These lettuce boats are a low-carb alternative to traditional sandwiches, offering a satisfying, protein-packed snack. The crisp lettuce adds a refreshing crunch, while the tuna salad provides creamy, flavorful filling.

Nutritional Benefits:

- **Tuna:** Provides high-quality protein and essential nutrients like omega-3 fatty acids.

- **Lettuce:** Low in calories and carbs, adding fiber and hydration.

Variations:

- **Tuna Variations:** Add chopped pickles, olives, or herbs to the tuna salad for additional flavor.

- **Lettuce Alternatives:** Use other types of leafy greens like Swiss chard or collard greens.

9. Deviled Eggs

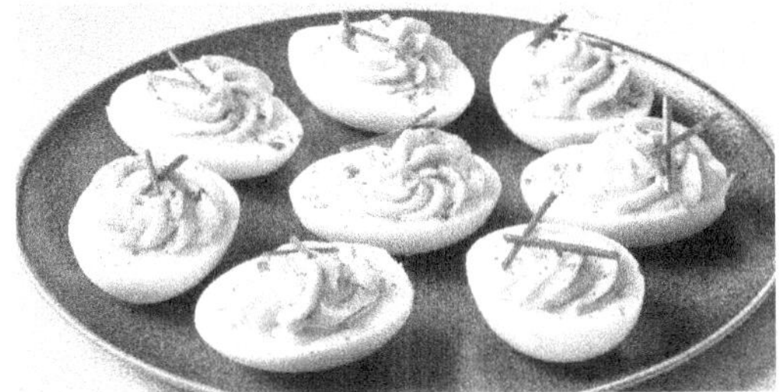

Description: Deviled eggs are a classic snack that combines the rich flavor of hard-boiled egg yolks with a creamy, seasoned filling. This snack is both nutritious and versatile, making it a great option for those seeking a high-protein, low-carb treat.

Ingredients:

- **6 hard-boiled eggs:** Cooked, peeled, and halved.

- **1/4 cup mayonnaise:** Use a low-carb version if desired.

- **1 teaspoon Dijon mustard:** Adds a tangy flavor.

- **1 tablespoon chopped pickles or relish:** For added crunch and flavor.

- **Paprika for garnish**

- **Salt and pepper to taste**

Instructions:

1. **Prepare the Eggs:** Halve the hard-boiled eggs and remove the yolks.

2. **Mix the Filling:** Mash the yolks with mayonnaise, mustard, pickles, salt, and pepper until smooth.

3. **Stuff the Eggs:** Spoon or pipe the yolk mixture back into the egg whites.

4. **Garnish and Serve:** Sprinkle with paprika and serve.

Why It's Great: Deviled eggs offer a rich, creamy snack that is high in protein and low in carbohydrates. They are easy to prepare and can be made in advance, making them a great option for quick snacks or gatherings.

Nutritional Benefits:

- **Eggs:** High in protein, vitamins, and minerals, supporting overall health and satiety.

- **Mayonnaise and Mustard:** Add flavor without significant carbs.

Variations:

- **Flavor Add-ins:** Try adding ingredients like bacon bits, chives, or Sriracha for different flavor profiles.

- **Low-Fat Options:** Use Greek yogurt instead of mayonnaise for a lighter version.

10. Roasted Pumpkin Seeds

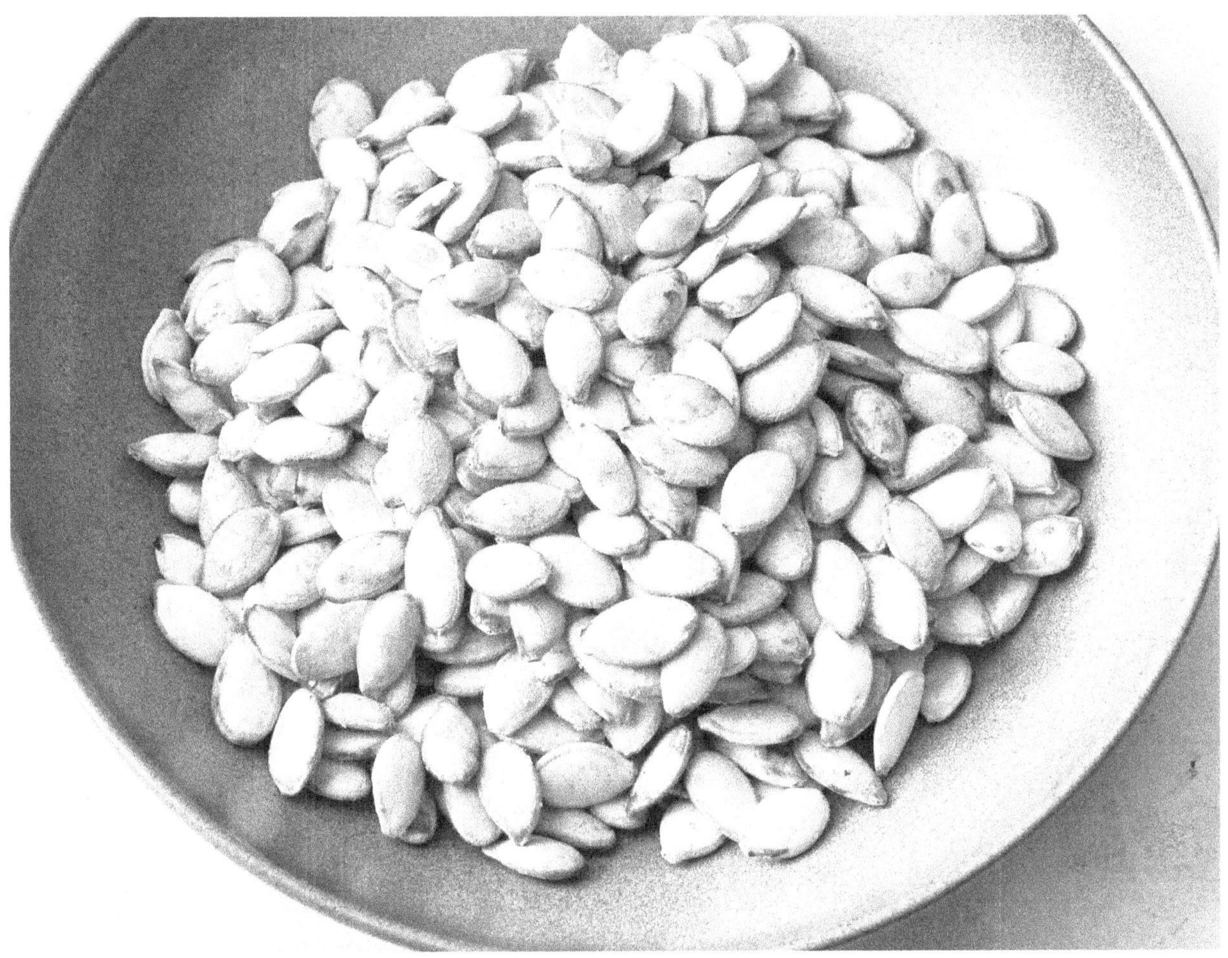

Description: Roasted pumpkin seeds are a crunchy, savory snack that's both nutritious and satisfying. These seeds are rich in protein, healthy fats, and essential minerals, making them a great choice for a nutrient-dense snack.

Ingredients:

- **1 cup pumpkin seeds:** Cleaned and dried.

- **1 tablespoon olive oil:** Helps to crisp the seeds.

- **1/2 teaspoon sea salt:** For seasoning.

- **Optional:** 1/2 teaspoon paprika or other spices for added flavor.

Instructions:

1. **Preheat Oven:** Set your oven to 350°F (175°C).

2. **Prepare the Seeds:** Toss pumpkin seeds with olive oil, salt, and any additional spices.

3. **Roast the Seeds:** Spread seeds in a single layer on a baking sheet.

4. **Bake:** Roast for 15-20 minutes, stirring occasionally, until golden brown and crispy.

5. **Cool and Serve:** Allow to cool before serving.

Why It's Great: Roasted pumpkin seeds are a crunchy, satisfying snack that provides a good source of protein and healthy fats. They are easy to make and can be seasoned to your liking, making them a versatile option for snacking.

Nutritional Benefits:

- **Pumpkin Seeds:** Rich in protein, magnesium, zinc, and healthy fats. They support heart health and provide a satisfying crunch.

Variations:

- **Seasoning Options:** Experiment with different spices like garlic powder, curry powder, or cayenne pepper.

- **Sweet Version:** For a different twist, try roasting with a touch of cinnamon and a small amount of sweetener.

These snack ideas are designed to be both nutritious and satisfying, helping you maintain stable blood sugar levels while providing a variety of flavors and textures. Each snack is low in carbs and high in essential nutrients, making them ideal for anyone looking to manage their diabetes effectively while enjoying delicious and wholesome snacks.

CHAPTER 6

DESSERTS

When following a low-carb, low-sugar diet, finding satisfying desserts can be challenging. These recipes offer a range of delicious, diabetes-friendly options that cater to various tastes while helping you stay within your dietary goals. Each dessert is crafted to provide both indulgence and nutritional balance, ensuring you enjoy a sweet treat without compromising your health.

1. Chia Seed Pudding

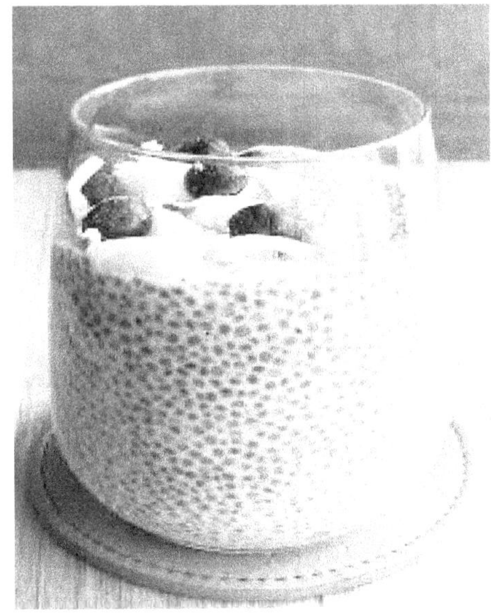

Description: Chia Seed Pudding is a versatile and nutritious dessert made from chia seeds soaked in a liquid, typically almond milk, until they form a pudding-like consistency. This dessert is rich in fiber, omega-3 fatty acids, and protein, making it a healthy choice that also satisfies your sweet tooth.

Ingredients:

- **1/4 cup chia seeds:** Packed with fiber and omega-3s.

- **1 cup unsweetened almond milk:** A low-carb milk alternative.

- **2 tablespoons chia seed sweetener (such as stevia or erythritol):** To add sweetness without carbs.

- **1 teaspoon vanilla extract:** For flavor.

- **Optional toppings:** Fresh berries, nuts, or a sprinkle of cinnamon.

Instructions:

1. **Mix Ingredients:** In a bowl, combine chia seeds, almond milk, sweetener, and vanilla extract. Stir well to ensure the chia seeds are evenly distributed.

2. **Refrigerate:** Cover the bowl and refrigerate for at least 2 hours or overnight. The chia seeds will absorb the liquid and expand, forming a pudding-like texture.

3. **Serve:** Stir the pudding before serving and add your favorite toppings if desired.

Why It's Great: Chia Seed Pudding is an easy-to-make dessert that provides a satisfying texture and rich flavor. It's high in fiber and omega-3s, promoting digestive health and satiety.

Nutritional Benefits:

- **Chia Seeds:** Provide essential fatty acids, fiber, and protein, which support heart health and digestion.

- **Almond Milk:** Low in carbs and calories, making it a suitable base for this dessert.

Variations:

- **Flavor Add-ins:** Experiment with different flavors by adding cocoa powder for a chocolate version or a touch of almond extract for a nutty twist.

- **Toppings:** Add a handful of fresh berries or a spoonful of unsweetened coconut flakes for extra flavor and texture.

2. Dark Chocolate and Almond Bark

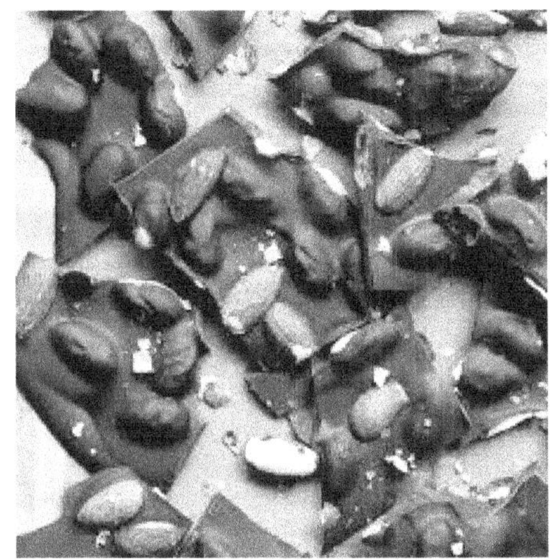

Description: Dark Chocolate and Almond Bark is a simple yet indulgent treat made with rich dark chocolate and crunchy almonds. This dessert is perfect for satisfying chocolate cravings while keeping the sugar content low.

Ingredients:

- **1 cup dark chocolate chips (85% cocoa or higher):** Choose high-quality chocolate with minimal sugar.

- **1/2 cup almonds (sliced or chopped):** Adds crunch and a nutty flavor.

- **1 tablespoon coconut oil:** Helps to smooth the chocolate.

Instructions:

1. **Melt the Chocolate:** In a heatproof bowl, melt the dark chocolate chips with coconut oil over a pot of simmering water (double boiler method) or in the microwave in 30-second intervals, stirring frequently.

2. **Prepare the Bark:** Line a baking sheet with parchment paper. Pour the melted chocolate onto the sheet and spread it into an even layer.

3. **Add Almonds:** Sprinkle chopped almonds over the melted chocolate, pressing them lightly into the surface.

4. **Chill:** Refrigerate until the chocolate is fully set (about 1 hour).

5. **Break and Serve:** Once set, break the bark into pieces and serve.

Why It's Great: This dark chocolate bark is a low-sugar treat that combines the richness of dark chocolate with the crunch of almonds. It's a great way to enjoy a sweet, satisfying dessert while keeping carbs and sugar levels in check.

Nutritional Benefits:

- **Dark Chocolate:** High in antioxidants and lower in sugar compared to milk chocolate.

- **Almonds:** Provide healthy fats, protein, and fiber.

Variations:

- **Add-ins:** Include other nuts like walnuts or pistachios, or sprinkle a small amount of sea salt on top for added flavor.

- **Flavored Chocolate:** Use chocolate with added flavors like orange or mint for a unique twist.

3. Keto Cheesecake Bites

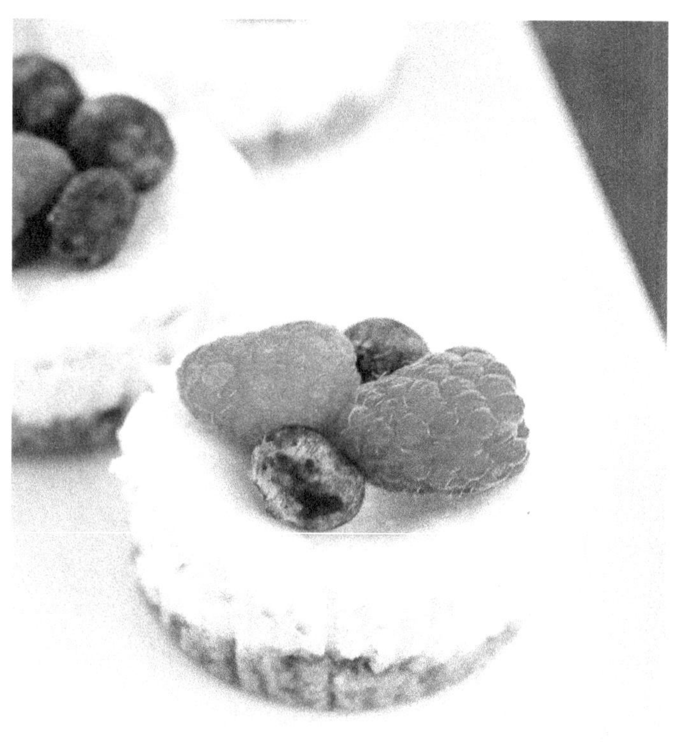

Description: Keto Cheesecake Bites are bite-sized, creamy treats that offer all the richness of traditional cheesecake without the carbs. These mini cheesecakes are perfect for portion control and are a great way to satisfy your sweet cravings.

Ingredients:

- **1 cup cream cheese:** Softened, for a creamy texture.

- **1/4 cup erythritol or another low-carb sweetener:** For sweetness without sugar.

- **1 teaspoon vanilla extract:** Adds flavor.

- **1 large egg:** Binds the mixture.

- **Optional crust:** 1/2 cup almond flour mixed with 2 tablespoons melted butter.

Instructions:

1. **Preheat Oven:** Preheat your oven to 325°F (163°C).

2. **Mix Ingredients:** In a bowl, beat together cream cheese, sweetener, vanilla extract, and egg until smooth.

3. **Prepare the Crust (Optional):** If using a crust, mix almond flour and melted butter, then press into the bottom of mini muffin cups.

4. **Fill and Bake:** Spoon the cheesecake mixture into mini muffin cups or a mini cheesecake pan.

5. **Bake:** Bake for 15-20 minutes or until set. Let cool before removing from the pan.

6. **Chill:** Refrigerate for at least 2 hours before serving.

Why It's Great: These cheesecake bites offer a creamy, indulgent dessert that fits perfectly into a keto diet. They are easy to make and provide a sweet treat without the high carb content of traditional cheesecake.

Nutritional Benefits:

- **Cream Cheese:** Provides a rich, creamy texture with minimal carbs.

- **Sweetener:** Low-carb sweeteners help keep blood sugar levels stable.

Variations:

- **Flavor Add-ins:** Add a bit of lemon zest, cocoa powder, or fresh berries to the cheesecake mixture for different flavors.

- **Toppings:** Top with a dollop of whipped cream or a drizzle of sugar-free chocolate sauce.

4. Sugar-Free Gelatin with Whipped Cream

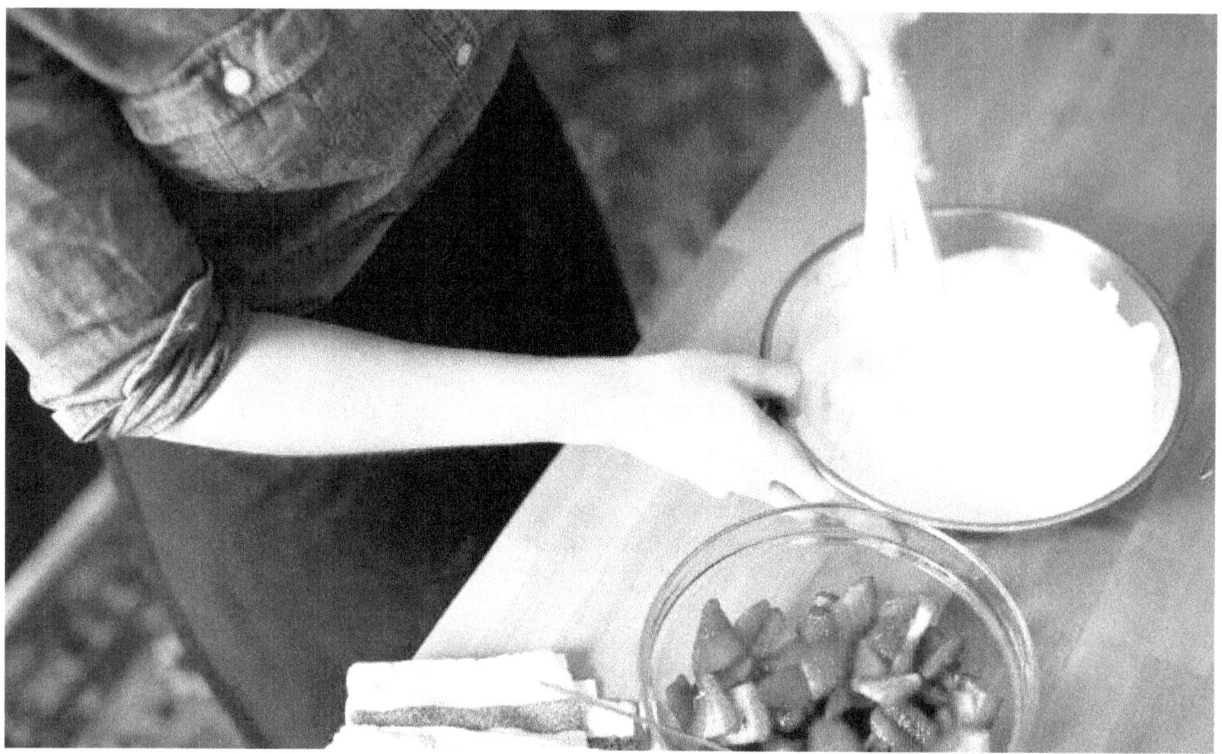

Description: Sugar-Free Gelatin with Whipped Cream is a light and refreshing dessert that's quick to prepare and perfect for those who enjoy a sweet yet guilt-free treat. This dessert combines the fruity flavors of sugar-free gelatin with a dollop of homemade whipped cream.

Ingredients:

- **1 package sugar-free gelatin:** Choose your favorite flavor.

- **1 cup heavy cream:** For making the whipped cream.

- **2 tablespoons powdered erythritol or another low-carb sweetener:** Sweetens the whipped cream.

Instructions:

1. **Prepare the Gelatin:** Follow the package instructions to prepare the sugar-free gelatin. Pour into serving dishes and refrigerate until set.

2. **Make Whipped Cream:** In a bowl, whip heavy cream with a mixer until it forms soft peaks. Add sweetener to taste.

3. **Serve:** Spoon whipped cream over the set gelatin before serving.

Why It's Great: This dessert is light and easy to make, offering a refreshing and satisfying option for those on a low-carb diet. The combination of gelatin and whipped cream provides a sweet and creamy treat without the sugar.

Nutritional Benefits:

- **Gelatin:** Low in calories and carbs, providing a sweet taste without sugar.

- **Heavy Cream:** Adds richness and is low in carbs, especially when sweetened with a low-carb sweetener.

Variations:

- **Flavor Combinations:** Use different flavors of sugar-free gelatin and add fresh berries or a splash of vanilla extract to the whipped cream.

- **Gelatin Shapes:** For a fun twist, use gelatin molds to create different shapes.

5. Coconut Macaroons

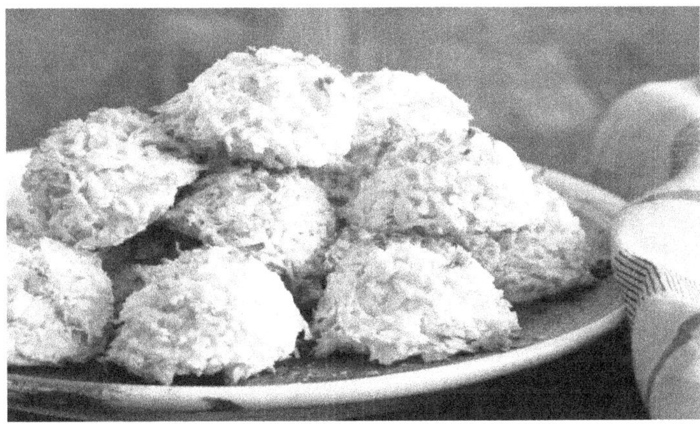

Description: Coconut Macaroons are sweet, chewy treats made with shredded coconut and often dipped in dark chocolate. These macaroons are naturally low in carbs and provide a delicious, chewy texture with a hint of tropical flavor.

Ingredients:

- **2 cups shredded unsweetened coconut:** Provides the chewy texture.

- **1/2 cup egg whites:** Helps bind the coconut.

- **1/4 cup erythritol or other low-carb sweetener:** Adds sweetness.

- **1/2 teaspoon vanilla extract:** For flavor.

- **Optional:** 1/2 cup dark chocolate chips for dipping.

Instructions:

1. **Preheat Oven:** Preheat your oven to 325°F (163°C) and line a baking sheet with parchment paper.

2. **Mix Ingredients:** In a bowl, combine shredded coconut, egg whites, sweetener, and vanilla extract. Mix well.

3. **Form Macaroons:** Spoon small mounds of the mixture onto the prepared baking sheet.

4. **Bake:** Bake for 15-20 minutes or until the edges are golden brown.

5. **Cool and Optional Chocolate Dip:** Let cool. If desired, melt dark chocolate and dip the bottom of each macaroon into the chocolate, then refrigerate until set.

Why It's Great: Coconut Macaroons are a deliciously sweet treat that's naturally low in carbs and high in fiber. They are easy to make and can be customized with a chocolate dip for added indulgence.

Nutritional Benefits:

- **Shredded Coconut:** Provides fiber and healthy fats.

- **Egg Whites:** Offer a source of protein.

Variations:

- **Flavored Macaroons:** Add a few drops of almond extract or citrus zest for a different flavor.

- **Chocolate Options:** Use sugar-free dark chocolate or drizzle with melted chocolate for a decadent touch.

6. Low Carb Lemon Bars

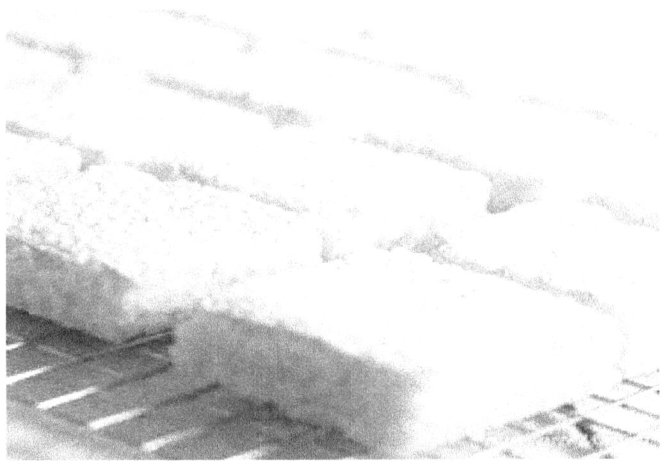

Description: Low Carb Lemon Bars are a tangy and refreshing dessert that delivers the bright, zesty flavor of lemon with a reduced sugar content. The crust and filling are made with low-carb ingredients, making these bars a delightful treat that fits your dietary needs.

Ingredients:

- **For the Crust:**
    - **1 cup almond flour**
    - **1/4 cup butter, melted**
    - **2 tablespoons erythritol or other low-carb sweetener**

- **For the Filling:**

  - 1/2 cup lemon juice (freshly squeezed)

  - 1/4 cup erythritol or other low-carb sweetener

  - 3 large eggs

  - 1/4 cup coconut flour

  - 1/4 teaspoon baking powder

  - 1/4 teaspoon vanilla extract

Instructions:

1. **Preheat Oven:** Preheat your oven to 350°F (175°C) and line an 8x8 inch baking pan with parchment paper.

2. **Prepare the Crust:** Mix almond flour, melted butter, and sweetener in a bowl. Press the mixture into the bottom of the prepared pan.

3. **Bake Crust:** Bake for 10 minutes, then remove from the oven.

4. **Prepare the Filling:** In a separate bowl, whisk together lemon juice, sweetener, eggs, coconut flour, baking powder, and vanilla extract.

5. **Assemble and Bake:** Pour the lemon filling over the pre-baked crust. Return to the oven and bake for an additional 20-25 minutes, or until the filling is set and slightly golden.

6. **Cool and Slice:** Allow to cool completely before cutting into bars.

Why It's Great: These lemon bars are a tart and sweet treat that offers a refreshing burst of citrus flavor while keeping carbs to a minimum. They are perfect for a light, satisfying dessert.

Nutritional Benefits:

- **Lemon Juice:** Provides a good source of vitamin C and adds a refreshing flavor.

- **Almond Flour and Coconut Flour:** Offer low-carb alternatives to traditional flour.

Variations:

- **Berry Lemon Bars:** Add a layer of fresh berries on top of the filling before baking for a fruity twist.

- **Glazed Bars:** Drizzle with a sugar-free lemon glaze for extra sweetness.

7. Almond Flour Brownies

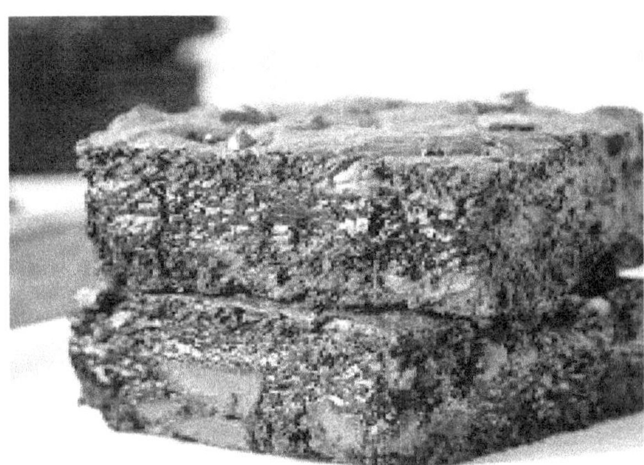

Description: Almond Flour Brownies are rich and fudgy treats that use almond flour as a low-carb substitute for traditional flour. These brownies are perfect for chocolate lovers seeking a gluten-free and lower-carb dessert option.

Ingredients:

- **1 cup almond flour**

- **1/2 cup unsweetened cocoa powder**

- **1/2 cup erythritol or another low-carb sweetener**

- **1/2 cup butter, melted**

- **2 large eggs**

- **1 teaspoon vanilla extract**

- **1/2 teaspoon baking powder**

- **Optional: 1/2 cup sugar-free chocolate chips**

Instructions:

1. **Preheat Oven:** Preheat your oven to 350°F (175°C) and line an 8x8 inch baking pan with parchment paper.

2. **Mix Ingredients:** In a bowl, combine almond flour, cocoa powder, sweetener, and baking powder. Stir in melted butter, eggs, and vanilla extract until smooth.

3. **Add Chocolate Chips (Optional):** Fold in chocolate chips if using.

4. **Bake:** Pour the batter into the prepared pan and spread evenly. Bake for 20-25 minutes, or until a toothpick inserted into the center comes out mostly clean.

5. **Cool and Serve:** Allow to cool completely before cutting into squares.

Why It's Great: These almond flour brownies offer a rich, chocolatey experience with fewer carbs and gluten-free ingredients. They are ideal for satisfying a sweet tooth while staying within dietary constraints.

Nutritional Benefits:

- **Almond Flour:** Provides healthy fats, fiber, and protein.

- **Cocoa Powder:** Offers antioxidants and a rich chocolate flavor.

Variations:

- **Nut Add-ins:** Add chopped nuts or sugar-free chocolate chunks for extra texture.

- **Frosting:** Top with a low-carb chocolate or cream cheese frosting for added indulgence.

8. Berry Compote with Greek Yogurt

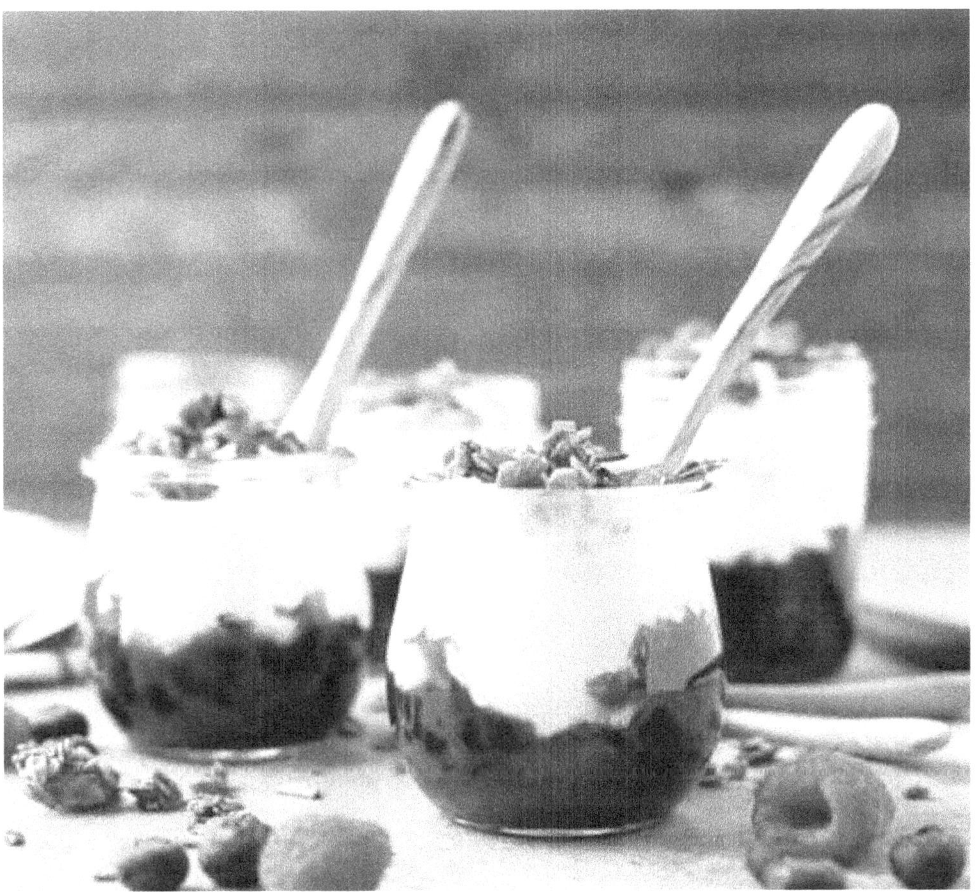

Description: Berry Compote with Greek Yogurt is a fresh and light dessert that combines a tangy yogurt base with a sweet and fruity berry compote. This dessert is rich in protein and antioxidants, making it a healthy choice for a satisfying treat.

Ingredients:

- **For the Berry Compote:**

- o **2 cups mixed berries (such as strawberries, blueberries, and raspberries)**

    - o **2 tablespoons erythritol or other low-carb sweetener**

    - o **1 tablespoon lemon juice**

- **For the Yogurt:**

    - o **1 cup Greek yogurt (plain, full-fat)**

    - o **1 teaspoon vanilla extract**

Instructions:

1. **Prepare the Compote:** In a saucepan, combine berries, sweetener, and lemon juice. Cook over medium heat, stirring occasionally, until the berries break down and the mixture thickens (about 10-15 minutes).

2. **Prepare the Yogurt:** In a bowl, mix Greek yogurt with vanilla extract.

3. **Assemble:** Spoon Greek yogurt into serving dishes and top with warm or chilled berry compote.

4. **Serve:** Enjoy immediately or chill in the refrigerator before serving.

Why It's Great: This dessert is both refreshing and nutritious, combining the protein-rich Greek yogurt with antioxidant-packed berries. It's an excellent choice for a quick and healthy dessert.

Nutritional Benefits:

- **Greek Yogurt:** High in protein and probiotics, supporting digestive health.

- **Berries:** Provide antioxidants, vitamins, and a burst of natural sweetness.

Variations:

- **Berry Combinations:** Use different types of berries or add a hint of cinnamon or nutmeg to the compote.

- **Yogurt Options:** Substitute Greek yogurt with a dairy-free alternative if preferred.

9. Chocolate Avocado Mousse

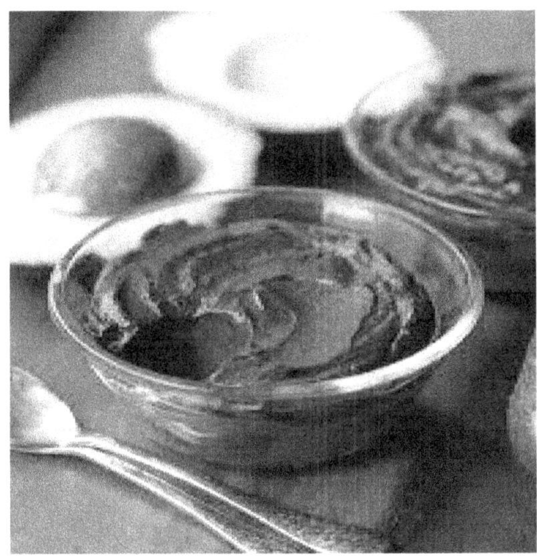

Description: Chocolate Avocado Mousse is a creamy and indulgent dessert that uses ripe avocados as a base for a rich chocolate mousse. This dessert is not only delicious but also packed with healthy fats and nutrients, making it a great choice for a low-carb diet.

Ingredients:

- **2 ripe avocados:** Provide a creamy base and healthy fats.

- **1/4 cup unsweetened cocoa powder:** Adds rich chocolate flavor.

- **1/4 cup erythritol or another low-carb sweetener:** For sweetness.

- **1/4 cup almond milk or coconut milk:** Helps to blend the ingredients.

- **1 teaspoon vanilla extract:** For added flavor.

Instructions:

1. **Prepare the Ingredients:** Scoop the flesh from the avocados and place in a blender or food processor.

2. **Blend:** Add cocoa powder, sweetener, almond milk, and vanilla extract. Blend until smooth and creamy.

3. **Chill:** Refrigerate for at least 30 minutes to allow the mousse to firm up.

4. **Serve:** Spoon into serving dishes and enjoy.

Why It's Great: This chocolate mousse offers a rich, creamy texture without the sugar or dairy of traditional desserts. It's a perfect way to enjoy a sweet treat while benefiting from the healthy fats in avocados.

Nutritional Benefits:

- **Avocados:** Provide healthy monounsaturated fats, fiber, and a range of vitamins and minerals.

- **Cocoa Powder:** Offers antioxidants and a rich chocolate flavor with minimal sugar.

Variations:

- **Flavor Add-ins:** Add a pinch of sea salt, a splash of coffee, or a few drops of mint extract for different flavor profiles.

- **Toppings:** Garnish with fresh berries, a dollop of whipped cream, or a sprinkle of chopped nuts.

10. Peanut Butter Fat Bombs

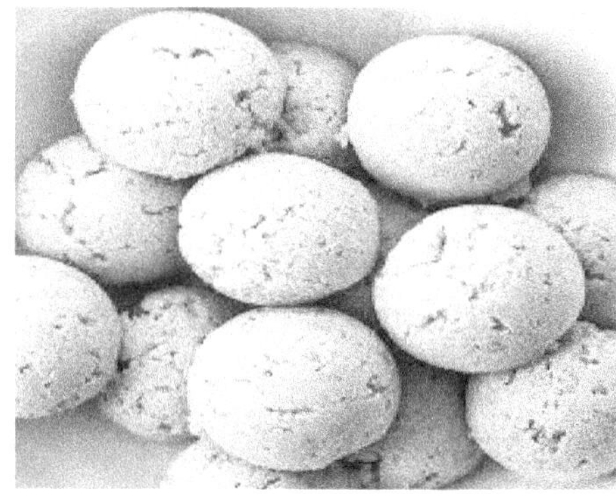

Description: Peanut Butter Fat Bombs are small, rich treats that are perfect for satisfying cravings while adhering to a low-carb diet. These fat bombs are made with peanut butter and healthy fats, making them a great snack or dessert option.

Ingredients:

- **1/2 cup peanut butter (natural, unsweetened):** Provides flavor and healthy fats.

- **1/4 cup coconut oil:** Adds healthy fats and helps solidify the bombs.

- **2 tablespoons erythritol or other low-carb sweetener:** For sweetness.

- **1/2 teaspoon vanilla extract:** Adds flavor.

Instructions:

1. **Mix Ingredients:** In a bowl, combine peanut butter, coconut oil, sweetener, and vanilla extract. Stir until well mixed.

2. **Form the Bombs:** Spoon the mixture into silicone molds or mini muffin cups.

3. **Chill:** Refrigerate until firm, about 30 minutes.

4. **Serve:** Pop out of molds and enjoy.

Why It's Great: These fat bombs are a great way to enjoy a rich, satisfying treat that's low in carbs and high in healthy fats. They're perfect for a quick snack or as a dessert to satisfy your cravings.

Nutritional Benefits:

- **Peanut Butter:** Provides protein and healthy fats, supporting satiety.

- **Coconut Oil:** Adds medium-chain triglycerides (MCTs) that are beneficial for energy and metabolism.

Variations:

- **Add-ins:** Mix in a few sugar-free chocolate chips or a sprinkle of sea salt for extra flavor.

- **Flavor Variations:** Use almond butter or cashew butter instead of peanut butter for different tastes.

These dessert options provide a variety of sweet treats that align with a low-carb lifestyle while still offering indulgent flavors and satisfying textures. Each recipe is crafted to deliver both taste and nutritional benefits, making them perfect for enjoying a dessert without compromising your dietary goals.

CHAPTER 7

MEAL PLANNING TIPS

Effective meal planning can make managing a diabetic diet more manageable and enjoyable. This section offers strategies and practical advice to help you stay organized, save time, and stick to your low sugar, low carb goals.

Creating a Weekly Meal Plan

Overview: A well-structured weekly meal plan is essential for maintaining a balanced diet, especially when managing diabetes. It helps ensure that you have nutritious, low-carb options readily available and reduces the likelihood of making impulsive food choices.

Steps to Create a Weekly Meal Plan:

1. **Assess Your Needs:**

    o **Nutritional Requirements:** Determine your daily calorie needs, macronutrient goals, and any specific dietary restrictions.

    o **Food Preferences:** Consider your taste preferences, and any food allergies or intolerances.

2. **Plan Your Meals:**

    o **Choose Your Recipes:** Select a variety of recipes that include breakfast, lunch, dinner, and snacks. Aim for recipes that use seasonal produce and incorporate a range of proteins, vegetables, and healthy fats.

    o **Balance Your Macronutrients:** Ensure each meal contains a balance of protein, fats, and low-carb vegetables to help stabilize blood sugar levels.

3. **Create a Shopping List:**

- o **List Ingredients:** Based on your meal plan, compile a list of all the ingredients you'll need. Group items by category (e.g., produce, dairy, meats) to make shopping easier.

  - o **Check Your Pantry:** Before heading to the store, check your pantry and fridge for items you might already have.

4. **Prepare for Flexibility:**

  - o **Substitute Ingredients:** Be prepared to swap out ingredients based on availability or personal preference.

  - o **Plan for Leftovers:** Include meals that can be repurposed or used as leftovers to save time and reduce waste.

5. **Schedule Your Cooking:**

  - o **Daily Prep:** Allocate time each day for meal preparation or cooking, considering your schedule and any busy periods.

  - o **Weekly Review:** Regularly review and adjust your meal plan based on what worked well and any changes in your dietary needs.

Why It's Great: Creating a weekly meal plan helps streamline grocery shopping, cooking, and ensures you're consistently eating balanced, diabetic-friendly meals. It can also reduce stress around meal times and minimize the temptation to grab unhealthy options.

Batch Cooking and Freezing

Overview: Batch cooking and freezing are time-saving strategies that can make it easier to stick to your meal plan, especially during busy weeks. Preparing meals in advance allows you to have healthy, low-carb options on hand at all times.

Steps for Batch Cooking:

1. **Choose Your Recipes:**

   - **Select Freezer-Friendly Recipes:** Opt for recipes that freeze well, such as soups, stews, casseroles, and baked dishes.

   - **Plan for Portion Sizes:** Cook in bulk and portion out meals into individual servings for convenience.

2. **Prepare Ingredients:**

   - **Pre-Cook Ingredients:** Cook proteins (like chicken, beef, or tofu) and vegetables in bulk. Use a slow cooker or pressure cooker to save time.

   - **Assemble Meals:** Combine ingredients for casseroles or bake dishes that can be easily frozen and reheated.

3. **Cool and Store:**

   - **Cool Properly:** Allow cooked food to cool to room temperature before freezing to prevent ice crystals from forming.

   - **Use Freezer Bags or Containers:** Store meals in airtight freezer bags or containers to avoid freezer burn. Label with the date and contents for easy identification.

4. **Reheat Safely:**

   - **Thawing:** Thaw frozen meals in the refrigerator overnight before reheating. For quick thawing, use the microwave's defrost function.

   - **Reheating:** Reheat meals in the oven, stovetop, or microwave, ensuring they reach an internal temperature of 165°F (74°C).

Why It's Great: Batch cooking and freezing help you maintain a healthy diet with minimal daily effort. It ensures you always have nutritious meals available, reducing the likelihood of reaching for unhealthy convenience foods.

Tips for Dining Out

Overview: Eating out while managing diabetes can be challenging, but with some strategic planning and knowledge, you can make healthier choices at restaurants.

Tips for Dining Out:

1. **Research the Menu:**

    - **Review Options Ahead of Time:** Look up the restaurant's menu online and choose dishes that align with your dietary goals.

    - **Ask for Modifications:** Don't hesitate to request modifications, such as substituting high-carb sides with vegetables or asking for sauces on the side.

2. **Make Smart Choices:**

    - **Focus on Protein and Vegetables:** Opt for meals that emphasize lean proteins and non-starchy vegetables. Avoid dishes that are breaded, fried, or covered in sugary sauces.

    - **Control Portions:** Choose smaller portions or share dishes to manage calorie intake.

3. **Watch Your Drinks:**

    - **Stick to Water or Unsweetened Beverages:** Avoid sugary drinks and limit alcohol consumption. Opt for water, unsweetened iced tea, or sparkling water.

4. **Be Mindful of Dressings and Sauces:**

    - **Request Dressings on the Side:** This allows you to control the amount used. Choose oil-based dressings over creamy ones.

- o **Be Cautious with Sauces:** Many sauces are high in sugar and carbs. Ask for them on the side or choose dishes without sauces.

5. **Plan Ahead:**

   - o **Eat a Small Snack Beforehand:** A small, healthy snack before dining out can help prevent overeating.

   - o **Understand the Nutritional Information:** Many restaurants provide nutritional information online or in-store. Use this to make informed decisions.

Why It's Great: These tips help you navigate dining out with confidence, ensuring you can enjoy meals with friends and family while sticking to your low-carb, diabetic-friendly diet.

Weekly Meal Plan Examples

Below are five sample weekly meal plans based on the recipes from this book. Each plan provides a variety of meals and snacks to keep your diet interesting and satisfying.

Sample Weekly Meal Plan 1:

- **Monday:**

  - o **Breakfast:** Avocado and Egg Breakfast Bowl

  - o **Lunch:** Grilled Chicken Salad with Avocado

  - o **Dinner:** Baked Salmon with Asparagus

  - o **Snack:** Almonds and Cheese

- **Tuesday:**

  - o **Breakfast:** Spinach and Feta Omelette

  - o **Lunch:** Zucchini Noodles with Pesto and Grilled Shrimp

- **Dinner:** Stuffed Bell Peppers with Ground Turkey

  - **Snack:** Cucumber Slices with Hummus

- **Wednesday:**

  - **Breakfast:** Low Carb Chia Seed Pudding

  - **Lunch:** Mediterranean Tuna Salad

  - **Dinner:** Garlic Butter Steak Bites with Green Beans

  - **Snack:** Celery Sticks with Peanut Butter

- **Thursday:**

  - **Breakfast:** Almond Flour Pancakes

  - **Lunch:** Spinach and Mushroom Stuffed Chicken Breast

  - **Dinner:** Lemon Herb Roasted Chicken with Brussels Sprouts

  - **Snack:** Hard-Boiled Eggs with a Dash of Hot Sauce

- **Friday:**

  - **Breakfast:** Breakfast Smoothie with Spinach and Protein Powder

  - **Lunch:** Cauliflower Rice with Stir-Fried Vegetables

  - **Dinner:** Shrimp Scampi with Zucchini Noodles

  - **Snack:** Greek Yogurt with Nuts and Seeds

- **Saturday:**

  - **Breakfast:** Cottage Cheese with Fresh Berries

  - **Lunch:** Turkey Lettuce Wraps

  - **Dinner:** Grilled Pork Chops with Cauliflower Mash

- o **Snack:** Guacamole with Veggie Sticks

- **Sunday:**

    - o **Breakfast:** Smoked Salmon and Avocado Toast on Low Carb Bread

    - o **Lunch:** Beef and Broccoli Stir-Fry

    - o **Dinner:** Eggplant Lasagna

    - o **Snack:** Deviled Eggs

Sample Weekly Meal Plan 2:

- **Monday:**

    - o **Breakfast:** Low Carb Breakfast Burrito with Turkey Sausage

    - o **Lunch:** Caprese Salad with Balsamic Glaze

    - o **Dinner:** Herb-Crusted Cod with Steamed Broccoli

    - o **Snack:** Roasted Pumpkin Seeds

- **Tuesday:**

    - o **Breakfast:** Greek Yogurt with Nuts and Seeds

    - o **Lunch:** Low Carb Chicken Caesar Wrap

    - o **Dinner:** Eggplant Lasagna

    - o **Snack:** Almonds and Cheese

- **Wednesday:**

    - o **Breakfast:** Coconut Flour Waffles

    - o **Lunch:** Grilled Chicken Salad with Avocado

- o **Dinner:** Baked Salmon with Asparagus

- o **Snack:** Celery Sticks with Peanut Butter

- **Thursday:**

  - o **Breakfast:** Breakfast Smoothie with Spinach and Protein Powder

  - o **Lunch:** Spinach and Mushroom Stuffed Chicken Breast

  - o **Dinner:** Garlic Butter Steak Bites with Green Beans

  - o **Snack:** Greek Yogurt with Nuts and Seeds

- **Friday:**

  - o **Breakfast:** Low Carb Chia Seed Pudding

  - o **Lunch:** Mediterranean Tuna Salad

  - o **Dinner:** Grilled Pork Chops with Cauliflower Mash

  - o **Snack:** Cucumber Slices with Hummus

- **Saturday:**

  - o **Breakfast:** Cottage Cheese with Fresh Berries

  - o **Lunch:** Cauliflower Rice with Stir-Fried Vegetables

  - o **Dinner:** Shrimp Scampi with Zucchini Noodles

  - o **Snack:** Guacamole with Veggie Sticks

- **Sunday:**

  - o **Breakfast:** Avocado and Egg Breakfast Bowl

  - o **Lunch:** Beef and Broccoli Stir-Fry

  - o **Dinner:** Stuffed Bell Peppers with Ground Turkey

- o **Snack:** Deviled Eggs

Sample Weekly Meal Plan 3:

- **Monday:**

  - o **Breakfast:** Spinach and Feta Omelette

  - o **Lunch:** Turkey Lettuce Wraps

  - o **Dinner:** Lemon Herb Roasted Chicken with Brussels Sprouts

  - o **Snack:** Greek Yogurt with Nuts and Seeds

- **Tuesday:**

  - o **Breakfast:** Almond Flour Pancakes

  - o **Lunch:** Mediterranean Tuna Salad

  - o **Dinner:** Zoodles with Meatballs in Marinara Sauce

  - o **Snack:** Roasted Pumpkin Seeds

- **Wednesday:**

  - o **Breakfast:** Coconut Flour Waffles

  - o **Lunch:** Low Carb Chicken Caesar Wrap

  - o **Dinner:** Baked Salmon with Asparagus

  - o **Snack:** Hard-Boiled Eggs with a Dash of Hot Sauce

- **Thursday:**

  - o **Breakfast:** Breakfast Smoothie with Spinach and Protein Powder

  - o **Lunch:** Spinach and Mushroom Stuffed Chicken Breast

  - o **Dinner:** Garlic Butter Steak Bites with Green Beans

- o **Snack:** Almonds and Cheese

- **Friday:**

    - o **Breakfast:** Low Carb Chia Seed Pudding

    - o **Lunch:** Cauliflower Rice with Stir-Fried Vegetables

    - o **Dinner:** Eggplant Lasagna

    - o **Snack:** Cucumber Slices with Hummus

- **Saturday:**

    - o **Breakfast:** Cottage Cheese with Fresh Berries

    - o **Lunch:** Grilled Chicken Salad with Avocado

    - o **Dinner:** Shrimp Scampi with Zucchini Noodles

    - o **Snack:** Celery Sticks with Peanut Butter

- **Sunday:**

    - o **Breakfast:** Greek Yogurt with Berries and Nuts

    - o **Lunch:** Beef and Broccoli Stir-Fry

    - o **Dinner:** Grilled Pork Chops with Cauliflower Mash

    - o **Snack:** Guacamole with Veggie Sticks

Sample Weekly Meal Plan 4:

- **Monday:**

    - o **Breakfast:** Avocado and Egg Breakfast Bowl

    - o **Lunch:** Zucchini Noodles with Pesto and Grilled Shrimp

    - o **Dinner:** Garlic Butter Steak Bites with Green Beans

- o **Snack:** Deviled Eggs

- **Tuesday:**

  - o **Breakfast:** Coconut Flour Waffles

  - o **Lunch:** Caprese Salad with Balsamic Glaze

  - o **Dinner:** Lemon Herb Roasted Chicken with Brussels Sprouts

  - o **Snack:** Greek Yogurt with Nuts and Seeds

- **Wednesday:**

  - o **Breakfast:** Low Carb Chia Seed Pudding

  - o **Lunch:** Turkey Lettuce Wraps

  - o **Dinner:** Baked Salmon with Asparagus

  - o **Snack:** Roasted Pumpkin Seeds

- **Thursday:**

  - o **Breakfast:** Spinach and Feta Omelette

  - o **Lunch:** Mediterranean Tuna Salad

  - o **Dinner:** Stuffed Bell Peppers with Ground Turkey

  - o **Snack:** Cucumber Slices with Hummus

- **Friday:**

  - o **Breakfast:** Almond Flour Pancakes

  - o **Lunch:** Low Carb Chicken Caesar Wrap

  - o **Dinner:** Shrimp Scampi with Zucchini Noodles

  - o **Snack:** Celery Sticks with Peanut Butter

- **Saturday:**

  - **Breakfast:** Greek Yogurt with Berries and Nuts

  - **Lunch:** Cauliflower Rice with Stir-Fried Vegetables

  - **Dinner:** Eggplant Lasagna

  - **Snack:** Guacamole with Veggie Sticks

- **Sunday:**

  - **Breakfast:** Breakfast Smoothie with Spinach and Protein Powder

  - **Lunch:** Spinach and Mushroom Stuffed Chicken Breast

  - **Dinner:** Grilled Pork Chops with Cauliflower Mash

  - **Snack:** Hard-Boiled Eggs with a Dash of Hot Sauce

Sample Weekly Meal Plan 5:

- **Monday:**

  - **Breakfast:** Low Carb Breakfast Burrito with Turkey Sausage

  - **Lunch:** Grilled Chicken Salad with Avocado

  - **Dinner:** Herb-Crusted Cod with Steamed Broccoli

  - **Snack:** Almonds and Cheese

- **Tuesday:**

  - **Breakfast:** Cottage Cheese with Fresh Berries

  - **Lunch:** Cauliflower Rice with Stir-Fried Vegetables

  - **Dinner:** Eggplant Lasagna

  - **Snack:** Greek Yogurt with Nuts and Seeds

- **Wednesday:**

    - o **Breakfast:** Coconut Flour Waffles

    - o **Lunch:** Mediterranean Tuna Salad

    - o **Dinner:** Grilled Pork Chops with Cauliflower Mash

    - o **Snack:** Celery Sticks with Peanut Butter

- **Thursday:**

    - o **Breakfast:** Spinach and Feta Omelette

    - o **Lunch:** Low Carb Chicken Caesar Wrap

    - o **Dinner:** Baked Salmon with Asparagus

    - o **Snack:** Guacamole with Veggie Sticks

- **Friday:**

    - o **Breakfast:** Avocado and Egg Breakfast Bowl

    - o **Lunch:** Beef and Broccoli Stir-Fry

    - o **Dinner:** Shrimp Scampi with Zucchini Noodles

    - o **Snack:** Cucumber Slices with Hummus

- **Saturday:**

    - o **Breakfast:** Greek Yogurt with Berries and Nuts

    - o **Lunch:** Spinach and Mushroom Stuffed Chicken Breast

    - o **Dinner:** Garlic Butter Steak Bites with Green Beans

    - o **Snack:** Roasted Pumpkin Seeds

- **Sunday:**

- **Breakfast:** Breakfast Smoothie with Spinach and Protein Powder

- **Lunch:** Cauliflower Rice with Stir-Fried Vegetables

- **Dinner:** Zoodles with Meatballs in Marinara Sauce

- **Snack:** Deviled Eggs

These meal plan examples incorporate a variety of recipes from the book, ensuring a diverse and satisfying weekly menu that aligns with your low sugar, low carb dietary goals.

GROCERY SHOPPING GUIDE

Navigating the grocery store with a focus on maintaining a low sugar, low carb diet can be overwhelming, especially with the variety of products available. This comprehensive guide will help you make informed choices, read nutrition labels effectively, and shop within your budget while sticking to your dietary goals.

Shopping for Low Sugar, Low Carb Ingredients

Overview: When shopping for a low sugar, low carb diet, it's essential to select ingredients that align with your nutritional goals. Focus on whole, unprocessed foods, and be mindful of hidden sugars and carbs in packaged products.

Key Strategies:

1. **Prioritize Whole Foods:**

   - **Fresh Vegetables:** Choose non-starchy vegetables like leafy greens, bell peppers, cucumbers, and zucchini. These are low in carbs and rich in essential nutrients.

   - **Proteins:** Opt for lean meats (chicken, turkey, fish), eggs, and plant-based proteins like tofu or tempeh. Check for added sugars or starches in processed meats.

   - **Healthy Fats:** Include sources like avocados, nuts, seeds, and olive oil. These provide healthy fats without added sugars.

2. **Avoid High-Carb Foods:**

   - **Grains:** Steer clear of bread, pasta, and rice, as they are high in carbohydrates. Look for low-carb alternatives like cauliflower rice or zucchini noodles.

- o **Sugary Snacks:** Avoid candies, pastries, and sugary beverages. Opt for snacks made with low-carb ingredients, such as nuts or cheese.

3. **Explore Low-Carb Alternatives:**

   - o **Flour Substitutes:** Use almond flour or coconut flour instead of wheat flour for baking.

   - o **Sweeteners:** Choose natural low-carb sweeteners like stevia or erythritol instead of sugar.

4. **Check for Hidden Sugars:**

   - o **Sauces and Dressings:** Many sauces and dressings contain hidden sugars. Look for options labeled "sugar-free" or "no added sugar."

   - o **Packaged Foods:** Be cautious with pre-packaged foods. Read labels carefully to avoid products with hidden sugars or high-carb ingredients.

Why It's Great: Shopping with a focus on low sugar and low carb ingredients ensures you are consuming foods that support your dietary goals, help manage blood sugar levels, and promote overall health.

Reading Nutrition Labels

Overview: Understanding how to read nutrition labels is crucial for managing a low sugar, low carb diet. Nutrition labels provide information on the content of foods and help you make healthier choices.

Key Aspects of Nutrition Labels:

1. **Check Serving Size:**

   - o **Serving Information:** Pay attention to the serving size at the top of the label, as all nutritional information is based on this amount.

Adjust the values if you consume more or less than the serving size.

2. **Review Total Carbohydrates:**

   o **Net Carbs:** Focus on the total carbohydrates listed and subtract fiber and certain sugar alcohols to calculate net carbs. Net carbs are the carbohydrates that impact blood sugar levels.

   o **Fiber:** Look for foods high in dietary fiber, as fiber can help reduce the net carb count.

3. **Monitor Sugar Content:**

   o **Total Sugars:** Watch the total sugar content and avoid products with high amounts of added sugars. Check the ingredient list for terms like high-fructose corn syrup or cane sugar.

   o **Added Sugars:** Prefer products with minimal or no added sugars. Aim for foods with natural sugars, such as fruits, which provide additional nutrients.

4. **Examine Ingredient List:**

   o **Ingredient Quality:** Look for whole, recognizable ingredients. Avoid products with long lists of chemical additives or artificial ingredients.

   o **Hidden Carbs:** Be cautious of ingredients like maltodextrin or dextrose, which can contribute to the carb count despite appearing as minor components.

5. **Check for Nutritional Fortification:**

   o **Added Nutrients:** Some products may be fortified with vitamins and minerals, which can be beneficial. However, prioritize whole foods for nutrient intake over fortified processed foods.

Why It's Great: Reading nutrition labels helps you make informed decisions about the foods you buy, ensuring that they meet your low sugar, low carb requirements and supporting your health and dietary goals.

Budget-Friendly Shopping Tips

Overview: Maintaining a low sugar, low carb diet can be done on a budget with strategic shopping and planning. Implementing these budget-friendly tips can help you save money without compromising your dietary goals.

Tips for Budget-Friendly Shopping:

1. **Plan Your Meals:**

   - **Weekly Meal Planning:** Create a meal plan for the week to reduce impulse buys and ensure you purchase only what you need.

   - **Shopping List:** Prepare a detailed shopping list based on your meal plan and stick to it to avoid unnecessary purchases.

2. **Buy in Bulk:**

   - **Non-Perishables:** Purchase non-perishable items like nuts, seeds, and canned vegetables in bulk to save money.

   - **Freezer-Friendly Items:** Buy meat and fish in larger quantities and freeze portions to extend shelf life and reduce costs.

3. **Utilize Store Brands:**

   - **Generic Brands:** Opt for store or generic brands for items like dairy, nuts, and frozen vegetables, which are often less expensive but similar in quality to name brands.

4. **Look for Sales and Discounts:**

   - **Weekly Flyers:** Check store flyers and online deals for discounts on items you frequently use.

- o **Coupons:** Use coupons for additional savings on items that fit within your dietary guidelines.

5. **Shop Seasonal and Local:**

   - o **Seasonal Produce:** Purchase fruits and vegetables that are in season, as they tend to be less expensive and fresher.

   - o **Local Markets:** Visit local farmers' markets for fresh, affordable produce and potentially lower prices on other staple items.

6. **Use Frozen and Canned Options:**

   - o **Frozen Vegetables:** Choose frozen vegetables as a cost-effective alternative to fresh ones, especially for out-of-season produce.

   - o **Canned Goods:** Opt for low-sodium canned vegetables or beans for budget-friendly options, and ensure they fit within your carb and sugar requirements.

7. **Grow Your Own:**

   - o **Herbs and Vegetables:** Consider growing your own herbs and low-carb vegetables, such as lettuce or spinach, to save money and ensure a fresh supply.

Why It's Great: Implementing these budget-friendly shopping tips allows you to manage costs while adhering to your low sugar, low carb diet. Efficient shopping strategies help you stay within your budget and make the most out of your grocery spending.

These comprehensive grocery shopping tips will help you make healthier choices, effectively read nutrition labels, and maintain a budget-friendly approach while adhering to a low sugar, low carb lifestyle.

ADDITIONAL RESOURCES

Navigating a low sugar, low carb diet while managing diabetes can be enhanced by leveraging additional resources. This section provides recommendations for books, websites, support groups, and apps that offer valuable information and support for your journey.

Recommended Books and Websites

Books:

1. **"The Diabetes Diet: Dr. Bernstein's Low-Carbohydrate Solution" by Richard K. Bernstein**

   - **Description:** This book provides a comprehensive guide to managing diabetes through a low-carb diet. Dr. Bernstein, a renowned diabetes specialist, shares his approach to controlling blood sugar levels with practical advice and recipes.

   - **Why It's Great:** Offers detailed strategies and meal plans for achieving stable blood sugar levels and improved health.

2. **"The Low-Carb Cookbook for Diabetics" by Katie Caldesi and Giancarlo Caldesi**

   - **Description:** This cookbook focuses on low-carb recipes tailored for diabetics. It includes a variety of delicious dishes designed to help manage blood sugar levels while enjoying flavorful meals.

   - **Why It's Great:** Provides practical, easy-to-follow recipes that align with diabetic dietary needs.

3. **"The Diabetes Code: Prevent and Reverse Type 2 Diabetes Naturally" by Dr. Jason Fung**

   - **Description:** Dr. Fung presents a holistic approach to reversing Type 2 diabetes through dietary changes, intermittent fasting, and lifestyle adjustments.

- o **Why It's Great:** Offers insights into the underlying causes of Type 2 diabetes and practical steps for managing and potentially reversing the condition.

4. **"The Complete Guide to Fasting: Heal Your Body Through Intermittent, Alternate-Day, and Extended Fasting" by Dr. Jason Fung and Jimmy Moore**

   - o **Description:** This guide explores various fasting methods and their benefits for metabolic health, including diabetes management.

   - o **Why It's Great:** Provides a comprehensive look at how fasting can be used as a tool for managing blood sugar and improving overall health.

5. **"Low-Carb Diet Cookbook for Beginners: 150 Simple and Delicious Recipes" by Sarah Johnson**

   - o **Description:** A cookbook designed for beginners with easy-to-make low-carb recipes that are ideal for managing diabetes.

   - o **Why It's Great:** Includes a range of recipes from breakfast to dinner, making it easier to stick to a low-carb diet.

Websites:

1. **American Diabetes Association (ADA) - www.diabetes.org**

   - o **Description:** A leading resource for diabetes information, including educational materials, research updates, and dietary recommendations.

   - o **Why It's Great:** Offers extensive resources on diabetes management, including recipes, meal plans, and tips for living with diabetes.

2. **Diabetes.co.uk - www.diabetes.co.uk**

- o **Description:** A UK-based website providing support, resources, and information on diabetes management, including forums and dietary advice.

  - o **Why It's Great:** Features a community forum where users can share experiences and advice, alongside valuable resources for managing diabetes.

3. **Low Carb USA -** www.lowcarbusa.org

  - o **Description:** A platform dedicated to promoting low-carb diets for managing diabetes and improving overall health. It includes articles, recipes, and event information.

  - o **Why It's Great:** Offers evidence-based information and a community focused on the benefits of low-carb living.

4. **NutritionFacts.org -** www.nutritionfacts.org

  - o **Description:** A website by Dr. Michael Greger providing research-based information on nutrition and health, including insights on managing diabetes.

  - o **Why It's Great:** Features videos and articles on the latest nutritional research and practical tips for healthier eating.

5. **The Low Carb Dietitian -** www.thelowcarbdietitian.com

  - o **Description:** A resource by dietitians specializing in low-carb diets, offering meal plans, recipes, and professional guidance.

  - o **Why It's Great:** Provides expert advice and practical tools for individuals seeking to follow a low-carb diet for health reasons.

Support Groups and Communities

Online Communities:

1. **Diabetes Daily Forums - www.diabetesdaily.com/forum**

- o **Description:** An online community where individuals with diabetes can connect, share experiences, and seek advice on managing their condition.

   - o **Why It's Great:** Offers peer support and practical tips from others who are managing diabetes.

2. **Reddit - r/diabetes -** www.reddit.com/r/diabetes

   - o **Description:** A subreddit dedicated to discussions about diabetes management, including diet, medication, and lifestyle tips.

   - o **Why It's Great:** Provides a platform for engaging discussions and advice from a diverse community of people with diabetes.

3. **Diabetes UK Online Community - www.diabetes.org.uk/forum**

   - o **Description:** A UK-based online forum offering support and advice for people living with diabetes, including a section for discussing diet and lifestyle.

   - o **Why It's Great:** Features a supportive community and resources specific to diabetes management.

4. **Facebook Groups - "Diabetes Support Group"**

   - o **Description:** Various Facebook groups dedicated to diabetes support, where members share their experiences, recipes, and tips.

   - o **Why It's Great:** Provides a sense of community and the opportunity to connect with others facing similar challenges.

5. **Type 1 Diabetes Support -** www.type1support.com

   - o **Description:** A support website for individuals with Type 1 diabetes, including forums, resources, and personal stories.

- o **Why It's Great:** Offers specialized support and resources tailored to Type 1 diabetes management.

Apps for Managing Diabetes and Meal Planning

Apps:

1. **MySugr - [Available on iOS and Android]**

   - o **Description:** A diabetes management app that allows users to track their blood sugar levels, medication, and food intake.

   - o **Why It's Great:** Provides a user-friendly interface and personalized insights to help manage diabetes effectively.

2. **Carb Manager - [Available on iOS and Android]**

   - o **Description:** An app designed for tracking carb intake, meal planning, and monitoring ketosis for those following a low-carb diet.

   - o **Why It's Great:** Helps with accurate tracking of carbs and provides meal suggestions aligned with low-carb goals.

3. **Glucose Buddy - [Available on iOS and Android]**

   - o **Description:** A comprehensive diabetes tracking app that allows users to log glucose levels, medication, and meals, and provides insights and reports.

   - o **Why It's Great:** Offers detailed tracking and analytical tools to manage diabetes more effectively.

4. **MyFitnessPal - [Available on iOS and Android]**

   - o **Description:** A popular app for tracking diet, exercise, and nutritional information. It supports users in managing their daily intake and achieving health goals.

- o **Why It's Great:** Provides extensive food databases and tracking features that are useful for monitoring carb and sugar intake.

5. **Fooducate - [Available on iOS and Android]**

   - o **Description:** An app that helps users make healthier food choices by scanning barcodes and providing nutritional information and healthier alternatives.

   - o **Why It's Great:** Offers educational insights on food choices and helps users understand the nutritional value of various products.

Utilizing these additional resources, including books, websites, support communities, and apps, can provide you with valuable information, support, and tools for managing diabetes and maintaining a low sugar, low carb diet. They offer a range of perspectives and practical advice to enhance your knowledge and improve your health journey.

CONCLUSION

As you reach the end of this guide, it's important to reflect on the journey you've undertaken and the path ahead. This conclusion aims to provide a succinct recap of the key points covered, offer encouragement, and share final thoughts to support you as you continue your journey toward better health and well-being.

Recap of Key Points

1. **Understanding Diabetes and Diet:**

   - **Diabetes Management:** Managing diabetes involves understanding how different foods affect blood sugar levels. Low sugar and low carb diets are crucial in controlling glucose levels and maintaining overall health.

   - **Meal Planning:** Effective meal planning is essential for adhering to a low sugar, low carb diet. By planning meals ahead, you can ensure a balanced intake of nutrients while avoiding high-carb, high-sugar foods.

2. **Essential Ingredients and Tools:**

   - **Pantry Staples:** Stocking up on low-carb essentials such as almond flour, chia seeds, and coconut oil will make it easier to prepare diabetic-friendly meals.

   - **Kitchen Tools:** Investing in tools like a spiralizer, food processor, and a good set of measuring spoons can simplify the cooking process and help you stick to your dietary goals.

3. **Recipe Sections:**

   - **Breakfast Recipes:** Starting your day with nutritious and low-carb options like Avocado and Egg Breakfast Bowl or Almond

Flour Pancakes can help stabilize blood sugar levels and provide lasting energy.

- **Lunch Recipes:** Incorporating meals such as Grilled Chicken Salad with Avocado and Zucchini Noodles with Pesto ensures you stay full and satisfied while managing your carbohydrate intake.

- **Dinner Recipes:** Dishes like Baked Salmon with Asparagus and Eggplant Lasagna offer delicious and low-carb options that are perfect for a balanced evening meal.

- **Snack Ideas:** Healthy snacks, including Almonds and Cheese or Greek Yogurt with Nuts and Seeds, can help curb cravings and keep you on track throughout the day.

- **Desserts:** Enjoying treats like Chia Seed Pudding and Keto Cheesecake Bites can satisfy your sweet tooth without compromising your diet.

4. **Meal Planning Tips:**

- **Weekly Meal Plans:** Structuring your week with planned meals and snacks can help you stay organized and make healthier choices. Examples provided offer practical ways to incorporate recipes into your daily routine.

- **Batch Cooking:** Preparing meals in advance and freezing portions can save time and ensure you always have healthy options available.

5. **Grocery Shopping Guide:**

- **Shopping Tips:** Understanding how to shop for low sugar, low carb ingredients, read nutrition labels, and manage your grocery budget effectively is key to maintaining your diet.

- ○ **Additional Resources:** Utilizing recommended books, websites, and apps can offer further support and insights as you manage your diabetes and dietary needs.

Encouragement for Your Journey

Embarking on a journey to manage diabetes through diet can be both challenging and rewarding. Remember, every step you take toward better health is a victory. It's important to stay motivated and focused on your goals. Celebrate your successes, no matter how small, and use any setbacks as learning opportunities. Consistency is key, and making gradual changes will lead to sustainable results.

Seek support from friends, family, and online communities if you ever feel overwhelmed. Engaging with others who share similar experiences can provide encouragement, practical advice, and a sense of camaraderie.

Final Thoughts

As you continue to navigate your path toward better health, keep in mind that managing diabetes through a low sugar, low carb diet is a lifelong commitment. By applying the knowledge and strategies outlined in this guide, you are well-equipped to make informed choices that support your health and well-being.

Your journey is unique, and there will be ups and downs along the way. Embrace each day with a positive outlook and remain committed to your goals. Remember, you have the tools, resources, and support to achieve a balanced and fulfilling lifestyle while managing your diabetes effectively.

Thank you for allowing this guide to be a part of your journey. Here's to your health, success, and continued progress!